NATIONAL CANCER INSTITUTE
AND
AMERICAN CANCER SOCIETY

NATIONAL CANCER INSTITUTE

AND

AMERICAN CANCER SOCIETY

Criminal Indifference to Cancer Prevention and Conflicts of Interest

Samuel S. Epstein, M.D.

Chairman, the Cancer Prevention Coalition
and
Emeritus Professor Environmental and Occupational Medicine
University of Illinois School of Public Health

To order additional copies of this book, contact:
Xlibris Corporation
1-888-795-4274
www.Xlibris.com
Orders@Xlibris.com
97553

CONTENTS

NATIONAL CANCER INSTITUTE

AMERICAN CANCER SOCIETY

To my wondrous wife, Catherine,
who continues to make all things possible.

BIOGRAPHY OF THE AUTHOR

Leading International Authority on the Causes and Prevention of Cancer and on Cancer Policy

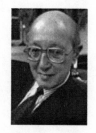

Samuel S. Epstein, MD, is professor emeritus of Environmental and Occupational Medicine at the University of Illinois School of Public Health and chairman of the Cancer Prevention Coalition. He has published some 270 peer-reviewed articles and authored or coauthored 20 books including the prize-winning 1978 *The Politics of Cancer*; the 1995 *Safe Shopper's Bible*; the 1998 *Breast Cancer Prevention Program*; the 1998 *The Politics of Cancer, Revisited*; the 2001 *GOT (Genetically Engineered) MILK! The Monsanto rBGH/BST Milk Wars Handbook*; the 2001 *Unreasonable Risk. How to Avoid Cancer from Cosmetics and Personal Care Products: The Neways Story*; the 2005 *Cancer-Gate: How to Win the Losing Cancer War*; the 2006 *What's in Your Milk?*; and the 2010 *Healthy Beauty*.

Dr. Epstein is an internationally recognized authority on avoidable causes of cancer, particularly unknowing exposures to industrial carcinogens in air, water, the workplace, and consumer products—food, cosmetics and toiletries, and household products including pesticides—besides carcinogenic prescription drugs.

Dr. Epstein's past public policy activities include serving as consultant to the U.S. Senate Committee on Public Works; drafting congressional legislation; having frequent invitation to congressional testimony; membership to key federal committees including EPA's Health Effects Advisory Committee and the Department of Labor's Advisory Committee on the Regulation of Occupational Carcinogens; and as key expert on banning of hazardous products and pesticides including DDT, aldrin, and chlordane. He is the leading international expert on cancer risks of petrochemicals and of consumer products including rBGH milk, meat from cattle implanted with sex hormones in feedlots on which he has testified for the EC at the January 1997 WTO hearings, and irradiated food. In 1998, he presented "Legislative Proposals for Reversing the Cancer Epidemic" to the Swedish Parliament and, in 1999, to the UK All Parliamentary Cancer Group. He has also submitted eight citizen petitions to the U.S. Food and Drug Administration on the undisclosed dangers of talc, lindane, nitrite-preserved foods, silicone gel and polyurethane implants, cosmetics containing DEA, rBGH, and hormonal beef.

He is also the leading critic of the cancer establishment, the National Cancer Institute (NCI) and American Cancer Society (ACS), for the fixation on damage control—screening, diagnosis and treatment, and genetic research—with indifference for cancer prevention, which, for the ACS, extends to hostility. This mind-set is compounded by ACS's conflicts of interest with the cancer drug industry and also with the petrochemical and other industries. The ACS thus qualifies for Ralph Nader's 1975 adage, "Jail for crime in the streets, [but] bail for crime in the suites."

Dr. Epstein's past professional society involvement includes being founder of the Environmental Mutagen Society, president of the Society for Occupational and Environmental Health, president of the Rachel Carson Council, and advisor to environmental, citizen activist, and organized labor groups.

His numerous honors include the 1969 Society of Toxicology Achievement Award; the 1977 National Wildlife Federation Conservancy Award; the 1989 Environmental Justice Award; the 1998 Right Livelihood Award (Alternative Nobel Prize) for international contributions to cancer prevention; the 1999 Bioneers Award; the 2000 Project Censored Award (Alternative Pulitzer Prize for investigative journalism) for an article critiquing the American Cancer Society; the 2005 Albert Schweitzer Golden Grand Medal for Humanitarianism from the Polish Academy of Medicine; and the 2007 Dragonfly Award from Beyond Pesticides.

Dr. Epstein has extensive media experience with numerous regional and national radio programs, including NPR; major TV programs, including *60 Minutes, Face the Nation, Meet the Press, The McNeil/Lehrer NewsHour, Donohue, Good Morning America,* and the *Today Show;* and Canadian, European, Australian, and Japanese TV. He has also contributed numerous editorials and letters to leading national newspapers and has published over 145 press releases and over 35 *Huffington Post* blogs over the last two decades.

ACKNOWLEDGMENTS

Warm commendations are due to Congressman John Conyers, Jr., chairman of the House Judiciary Committee, for his 1979 invitation to draft legislation on "white-collar crime" in relation to industry malpractice, knowingly exposing millions of citizens and workers to avoidable risks of cancer from industrial chemicals, and for his long-standing legislative initiatives on cancer policy; and to Dr. Quentin D. Young, past president of the American Public Health Association and now chairman of the Health and Medicine Policy Research Group, for their emphasis on the critical, but infrequently exercised, role of physicians in public health policy on the causes and prevention of cancer.

It is also a pleasure to acknowledge the over one hundred leading scientific experts in cancer prevention and public health and the representatives of activist citizen groups who endorsed the Cancer Prevention Coalition's February 2003 report, "Stop Cancer before It Starts Campaign: How to Win the Losing War against Cancer." This report deals with a wide range of avoidable causes of cancer—including unlabeled carcinogenic ingredients in consumer products, particularly cosmetics and personal care products—and related public policy concerns.

Finally, many thanks to my research assistant, Alessandra Elder, for her creative support.

NATIONAL CANCER INSTITUTE

Losing the Winnable War against Cancer

ENDORSED BY

Quentin D. Young, MD
Chairman, Health and Medicine Policy Research Group
Illinois Public Health Advocate
Past President, American Public Health Association

THE LOSING CANCER WAR

In 1971, Congress passed the National Cancer Act. This was initiated and promoted by the American Cancer Society (ACS), the world's wealthiest nonprofit organization, with behind-the-scenes strong support from the National Cancer Institute (NCI). The ACS promised that the cancer war could be won, given an increase in NCI's funding.

Spurred on by a major media campaign and aggressively promoted by the ACS, President Richard Nixon embraced the National Cancer Act. He then launched the War against Cancer and increased NCI's 1971 budget from $150 to $220 million. He also gave the NCI unprecedented autonomy within the National Institutes of Health (NIH). However, the Act had unintended consequences. It authorized the president to appoint the director of the NCI and approve its budget, thus bypassing the director of the other twenty-six National Institutes of Health. The Act thus effectively insulated and politicized the NCI.

Since passage of the 1971 Act, the NCI and ACS have repeatedly reassured the nation, with a steady stream press releases, briefings, and media reports, claiming major progress in the cancer war. These included assurances of miracle breakthroughs in cancer treatment and also promises, in 1984 and 1986, that cancer mortality would be halved by 2000.

However, over the past 40 years and a 25-fold increase of NCI's 1971 budget from $220 million to the currently proposed $5.2 billion (table 1), we are now further away from winning the cancer war than when it was first declared. This is clearly evidenced by the escalating incidence of a wide range of cancers from 1975 to 2007 (table 2), particularly nonsmoking cancers (table 3). These dramatic increases are paradoxically paralleled by NCI's escalating budget from 1973 to 2007 (chart) and from $220 million in 1971 to the current $5.1 billion. Examples of a wide range of nonsmoking cancers and their avoidable causes, which still remain ignored by the NCI, are listed in table 4. Over the last decade, NCI's alleged prevention budget has decreased from 11.8% of its total budget in 2000 down to 4.5% of its current budget (table 5).

TABLE 1: ESCALATING BUDGET OF THE NCI

YEAR	BUDGET*
1971	$220 m (National Cancer Act)
1975	$690 m
1980	$1.0 b
1985	$1.2 b
1990	$1.7 b
1995	$2.1 b
2000	$3.3 b
2005	$4.8 b
2010	$5.1 b
2011 (proposed)	$5.2 b

* m = millions; b = billions

Note: Approximate 25-fold increase from 1971 to 2011

TABLE 2: SEER Age-Adjusted Incidence Rates for Major Cancer Sites, 1975 and 2008

SITE		1975	2008	% Change
Childhood: Overall (ages 0-14)		11.5	15.2	32.2
Childhood: Overall (ages 0-19)		12.9	17.3	34.1
Non-Hodgkin Lymphoma				
Overall		11.1	20.2	82.5
Male		12.9	24.7	91.3
Female		9.6	16.6	72.9
Myeloma		4.9	5.8	18.6
Acute Lymphocytic Leukemia:		0.9	1.5	58.1
Ovary: Overall		16.3	12.6	-22.7
<65		11.6	7.4	-36.3
>65		48.9	48.7	-0.4
Cervix and Uteri		14.8	6.6	
Female Breast: Overall		105.1	127.3	21.1
Premenopausal		40.6	45.0	10.7
Postmenopausal		273.8	342.7	25.2
Testes		3.7	5.9	57.9
Brain and Other Central Nervous System		5.9	6.5	11.3
Thyroid		4.9	13.0	167.6
Melanoma		7.9	22.5	185.4
Kidney and Renal Pelvis		7.1	15.4	117.4
Liver and Intrahepatic Bile Duct		2.6	7.3	177.7
Pancreas		11.8	12.4	4.9
Bladder: Overall		19.3	20.7	7.1
Male		34.4	36.4	6.0
Female		8.9	9.1	2.4
Colon and Rectum		59.5	44.3	-25.6
Prostate		94.0	153.0	62.8
Lung and Bronchus:	Overall	52.3	58.8	12.5
	Male	89.5	70.2	-21.6
	Female	24.5	50.5	106.0
All Sites:	Overall	400.4	463.4	15.7
	Male	466.8	530.8	13.7
	Female	365.8	416.3	13.8

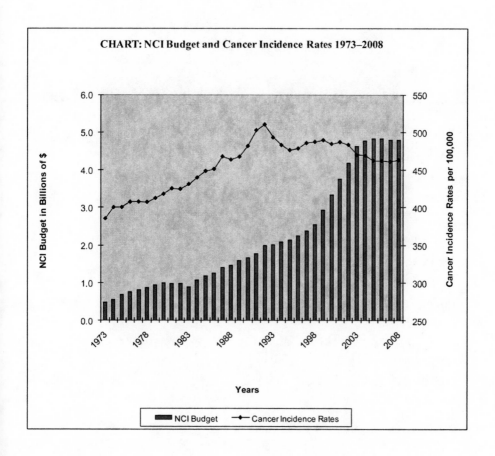

CHART: NCI Budget and Cancer Incidence Rates 1973–2008

TABLE 3: ESCALATING INCIDENCE OF NONSMOKING CANCERS

CANCER	% CHANGE 1975-2008
Multiple Myeloma	19
Postmenopausal Breast	25
Brain (childhood)	43
Testes	58
Acute Lymphocytic Leukemia (adult)	58
Acute Lymphocytic Leukemia (childhood)	63
Non-Hodgkin's Lymphoma	83
Kidney	117
Thyroid	168
Melanoma	185
Liver	178

TABLE 4: EXAMPLES OF THE INCREASING INCIDENCE OF NONSMOKING CANCERS AND THEIR AVOIDABLE CAUSES*

CANCER	% INCREASE IN INCIDENCE (1975-2008)	AVOIDABLE CAUSES
Malignant Melanoma	185	Use of sunscreens in childhood that fail to block long wave UV light
Thyroid	168	Ionizing radiation
Non-Hodgkin's Lymphoma	83	Phenoxy herbicides and phenylenediamine hair dyes
Acute Lymphocytic Childhood Leukemia	63	Ionizing radiation; domestic pesticides; nitrite preservatives in meats; parental exposures to occupational carcinogens
Testicular	58	Pesticides; hormonal ingredients in CPCP; estrogen residues in meat
Breast	21	Birth control pills; hormonal ingredients in CPCP; diagnostic radiation; routine premenopausal mammography
Ovary (mortality)	5.2 (black women)	Genital use of talc powder

*For further examples of avoidable causes of a wide range of cancers, see the President's Cancer Panel April 2010 Report (appendix F).

TABLE 5: NCI's CANCER PREVENTION BUDGET *

Year	Prevention $	Total Budget	Percent of Total Budget
2000	389,425,000	3.3 b	11.8%
2001	459,482,000	3.8 b	12.2%
2002	501,208,000	4.2 b	12.0%
2003	533,173,000	4.6 b	11.6%
2004	529,980,000	4.7 b	11.2%
2005	531,634,000	4.8 b	11.1%
2006	505,625,000	4.7 b	10.7%
2007	498,396,000	4.8 b	10.4%
2008	471,515,000	4.8 b	9.8%
2009	298,901,000	5.0 b	6.0%
2010	229,033,000	5.1 b	4.5%
2011	226,951,000 (proposed)	5.2 b	4.5%

* Based on NCI's Budget Analysis Interactive Tool

NCI'S IMBALANCED PRIORITIES

The research policies and priorities of the NCI remain dominated by professional mind-sets fixated on damage control—screening, diagnosis, chemoprevention, treatment—and treatment-related research. High priority for screening persists despite long-standing challenges as to its questionable effectiveness for cancers such as prostate, lung, premenopausal breast, and childhood neuroblastoma. Minimal emphasis, and even indifference, remains directed to the prevention of a wide range of avoidable causes of cancer—other than lifestyle factors, smoking, inactivity, and fatty diet—without consideration of carcinogenic contaminants.

In sharp contrast to predominant expenditures on treatment and related basic research, NCI's alleged prevention budget has been and remains minimal. A published, and unchallenged, analysis of its 1992 budget revealed that less than 2.5% of a $2 billion budget, in contrast to a claimed 20%, was allocated to research on avoidable carcinogens in air, water, food, the home, and the workplace.

In response to May 1998 questions by Congressman David Obey (D-WI), former NCI Director Klausner claimed that 20% of NCI's $2.5 billion budget was allocated to research on environmental causes of cancer. Following Obey's request for further information, Klausner failed to respond, other than increasing his previous estimate to 40%.

NCI's limited comprehension of prevention is revealed in the highlights of its 2001 Cancer Facts. The opening sentence states, "Cancer prevention is a major component and current priority—to reduce suffering and death from cancer." This was followed by the claim that 12% of NCI's $3.75 billion budget is allocated to prevention. However, this was explicitly defined in exclusionary terms of tobacco and faulty diet, without any reference to environmental and occupational carcinogens.

Not surprisingly, in February 2003, Congressman John Conyers (D-MI), ranking member of the House Judiciary Committee, warned that so much cancer carnage is preventable. "Preventable that is, if the NCI gets off the dime and does its job."

Failure to Inform the Public of Avoidable Risks of Cancer

With the exception of smoking and faulty diet, the NCI has failed to inform the public of published scientific information on a wide range of avoidable causes of multiple cancers—from involuntary and unknowing exposures to chemical and radioactive industrial carcinogens. These fall into three major categories: (1) environmental contaminants in air, water, soil, the workplace, and food; (2) carcinogenic ingredients in consumer products, particularly pesticides; (3) carcinogenic prescription drugs and high-dose diagnostic medical radiation, particularly pediatric CAT scans.

As critically, NCI has failed to inform Congress and regulatory agencies of such avoidable exposures to industrial and other carcinogens, incriminated in standard rodent tests and in epidemiological studies. Such information could have enabled the development of corrective legislative and regulatory action. This silence has also encouraged petrochemical and other industries to continue manufacturing carcinogenic products and corporate polluters to continue polluting unchallenged.

NCI's silence on cancer prevention is in flagrant violation of the 1971 National Cancer Act's specific charge "to disseminate cancer information to the public." This silence is in further violation of the 1988 Amendments to the National Cancer Program, which called for "an expanded and intensified research program for the prevention of cancer caused by occupational or environmental exposure to carcinogens."

Congressman David Obey also addressed the following question to NCI director Dr. Richard Klausner. "Should NCI develop a registry of avoidable carcinogens and make this information widely available to the public?" Dr. Klausner responded, "Such information is already available from NCI's Cancer Information Service." However, there is no basis whatsoever to support this claim.

NCI's silence on avoidable causes of cancer has even extended to suppression or denial of such information as illustrated by the following examples.

In 1983, the Department of Health and Human Services directed NCI to investigate the risks of thyroid cancer from I-131 radioactive fallout following atom bomb tests in Nevada in the late 1950s and early 1960s. NCI released its report in 1997, based on data which had been available for over fourteen years, predicting up to 210,000 thyroid cancers from radioactive fallout.

These cancers, whose incidence has almost doubled since 1973, could have been readily prevented had the NCI warned the public in time and advised them to take thyroid medication. At a September 1999 hearing by the Senate Subcommittee of the Committee on Government Affairs, former Senator John Glenn (D-OH) charged that the NCI investigation was "plagued by lack of public participation and openness." Senator Tom Harkin (D-IA) charged that NCI's conduct was a travesty.

As serious is NCI's frank suppression of information. At a 1996 San Francisco Town Hall Meeting on breast cancer, chaired by Congresswoman Nancy Pelosi (D-CA), former NCI director Richard Klausner insisted that "low level diagnostic radiation does not demonstrate an increased risk." However, this was contrary to long-term studies on patients with spinal curvature (scoliosis), which showed that such radiation was responsible for 70% excess breast cancer mortality.

The Public Remains Uninformed of Escalating Incidence of Childhood Cancer and Its Avoidable Causes

From 1975 to 2000, the incidence of childhood cancer has escalated to alarming proportions, warned the Cancer Prevention Coalition's in its May 2003 report, "The Stop Cancer before It Starts Campaign." Childhood cancers have increased by 32% overall to 9,000 annually: acute lymphocytic leukemia, 57%; brain cancer, 50%; kidney cancer, 48%; and bone cancer, 29%. Childhood cancer is their number one killer, with 1,500 deaths annually, second only to accidents.

The NCI and the American Cancer Society (ACS) have failed to inform the public of the increasing incidence of childhood cancer. Furthermore, the NCI claims that "the causes of childhood cancers are largely unknown." This is contrary to substantial scientific evidence on their avoidable causes, the wide range of carcinogens to which fetuses, infants, and children are exposed and their much greater vulnerability than adults. Additionally, most carcinogens cause other toxic effects hormonal or endocrine disruptive, neurological, and immunological.

Avoidable carcinogenic exposures of the fetus, infants, and children fall into three categories:

1. Environmental and Occupational

    -   Pesticides: contaminants in drinking water; urban spraying; uses in schools, including wood playground sets treated with chromated copper arsenate

- Petrochemical and other industrial pollutants: atmospheric emissions; contaminants in drinking water
- Combustion pollutants: power plants; incinerator stacks; diesel exhaust
- Radioactive pollutants: atmospheric emissions from nuclear energy plants; contaminants in drinking water
- Occupational carcinogens: parental exposures during pregnancy

2. Domestic/Household

- Pesticides: uses in the home, lawn, and pet flea collars; contaminants in nonorganic food
- Ingredients and contaminants in lotions and shampoos
- Residence near: hazardous waste sites; chemical and power plants; municipal incinerators

3. Medical

- Radiation: diagnostic X-rays in late pregnancy; high-dose radiation CAT scans of infants and children
- Pediatric prescription drugs: Lindane shampoos; Ritalin, for treatment of attention deficit disorder
- Drugs prescribed during pregnancy: the estrogenic DES; the antiepileptic Dilantin

NCI's silence on such causes of childhood cancer violates the charge of the 1971 National Cancer Act, launching President Nixon's War against Cancer "to disseminate cancer information to the public." This silence is also contrary to NCI's 1998 Congressional testimony that it had developed a public registry of avoidable carcinogens. Not surprisingly, the media remain as uninformed as the public. An April 1, 2003, *New York Times* article, "Success Stories Abound in Efforts to Prevent and Control Cancer," stated that while amazing progress has been made in treating childhood cancers, "their causes remain a mystery."

Besides the NCI silence on avoidable causes of childhood cancer, it has failed to provide scientific guidance to regulatory agencies as reflected in their inconsistent and questionable policies. This is illustrated in the well-intentioned current proposal of the Scientific Advisory Board of the Environmental Protection Agency to develop new guidelines for regulating risks from Early-Life Exposure to Carcinogens.

The minimal priorities of the NCI for research and providing the public with information on avoidable causes of childhood cancers reflect imbalanced policies and not lack of resources. NCI's annual budget has increased some 25-fold, from $200 million to $5.2 billion, since passage of the 1971 National Cancer Act. NCI expenditures on prevention of avoidable causes of cancer have been estimated as under 4% of its budget.

Exaggerated Claims of Progress in the War against Cancer

For over the last three decades, the NCI has made a series of highly publicized and misleading claims of major advances in the War against Cancer. These include the following:

- NCI's 1984 announcement, in its Cancer Prevention Awareness Program, that cancer mortality would be halved by 2000
- The same assurance in NCI's 1986 "Cancer Control Objectives" report
- The 1998 NCI and American Cancer Society (ACS) Report Card announcing a recent reversal of an almost twenty-year trend of increasing cancer incidence and deaths
- The February 2003 pledge by NCI director Andrew von Eschenbach, former ACS president-elect, to "eliminate the suffering and death from cancer by 2015"

In a September 2003 "Annual Report to the Nation on the Status of Cancer, 1975-2000," the NCI, ACS, and the Centers for Disease Control and Prevention claimed that "considerable progress has been made in reducing the burden of cancer in the U.S. population," particularly from 1995-2000; *burden* is defined as "the number of people with cancer." However, this claim is inconsistent with NCI's own data as detailed in its SEER Cancer Statistics Review, 1975-2000:

1975-2000 Statistics

- The overall cancer burden and incidence rates increased by 18%; rates for blacks increased by 20%.
- There has been a dramatic increase in the burden and incidence rates of a wide range of nonsmoking cancers. These include liver (104%); prostate (88%); non-Hodgkin's lymphoma (71%); thyroid (54%); testes (54%); breast (29%); acute myeloid leukemia (15%); and brain (14%). These increases have more than offset the 11% decline in lung cancer rates in men due to decreased smoking.

- The burden and incidence rates of childhood cancer have increased as follows: acute lymphocytic leukemia (59%); brain (48%); kidney (43%); and bone (20%).
- Overall cancer mortality rates have remained high (199 per 100,000) and unchanged; rates for blacks have increased by 6%.
- Mortality rates for prostate cancer, one of the major cancer killers, have decreased by only 1%.
- Mortality rates have increased by 46% for non-Hodgkin's lymphoma and 10% for brain cancer.

This increasing burden and incidence of cancer is in striking contrast to the 25-fold escalation of NCI's budget, from $220 million in 1971 to $4.6 billion in 2000. Paradoxically, it seems that the more we spend on cancer, the more cancer we get.

1995-2000 Statistics

- The overall burden and incidence rates remained virtually unchanged, decreasing by under 1%.
- There have been major increases in incidence rates of the following cancers: childhood kidney (43%); testes (24%); thyroid (19%); prostate (5%); acute myeloid leukemia (5%); brain (3%); and breast (2%).
- Mortality rates decreased as follows: overall (5%); prostate (18%); breast (13%); colorectal (8%); non-Hodgkin's lymphoma (6%); brain (4%); and lung (4%). This reflects improved diagnosis, treatment, and longer survival.

CONFLICTS OF INTEREST

NCI Leadership Conflicts of Interest and a Revolving Door with Industry

Benno C. Schmidt, the first chairman of President Nixon's 1971 three-member NCI Executive Cancer Panel, was an investment banker and senior drug company executive, with close ties to oil, steel, and chemical industries. He was followed in the 1980s by Armand Hammer, the late oil magnate and chairman of Occidental Petroleum, one of the nation's largest manufacturers of industrial chemicals, with major responsibility for the Love Canal disaster. Schmidt and Hammer showed no interest in cancer prevention. Instead, they focused on the highly profitable development and marketing of cancer drugs.

The late Dr. Frank Rauscher, appointed NCI director by President Nixon in 1971 to spearhead his War on Cancer, resigned in 1976 to become senior vice president of the ACS. In 1988, he moved on to become executive director of the Thermal Insulation Manufacturers Association, which promoted the use of carcinogenic fiberglass and fights against its regulation.

A 1993 analysis of conflicts of interest by board members of NCI's Memorial Sloan-Kettering Comprehensive Cancer Center revealed extensive ties to cancer drug companies, and oil, steel, fiberglass, and even tobacco industries, apart from $4 million institutional holdings in drug companies.

Dr. Samuel Broder, NCI director from 1989 to 1995, frankly admitted, in a 1998 *Washington Post* interview, that "the NCI has become what amounts to a government pharmaceutical company." Taxpayers have funded R & D and expensive clinical trials for over two-thirds of cancer drugs on the market. These drugs are then given, with exclusive rights, to the industry, which sells them at inflated prices. Broder resigned from the NCI to become chief scientific officer of Ivax and, later, chief medical officer of Celera Genomics; both are major manufacturers of cancer drugs.

Dr. Vincent DeVita, NCI director from 1980 to 1988, and Dr. John Mendelsohn, president of NCI's University of Texas MD Anderson Comprehensive Cancer Center, were both consultants and board members of ImClone Systems Inc. which had been seeking FDA approval of its targeted cancer drug, Erbitux. Neither DeVita nor Mendelsohn disclosed these interests in media interviews promoting targeted cancer drugs.

In October 2002, DeVita published an article, "The War on Cancer," in the *Cancer Journal* of which he is coeditor, claiming major progress in cancer drug treatment. However, he failed to disclose his commercial interests in targeted drugs and in his CancerSource.com website. This is contrary to the *Journal*'s disclaimer: "No benefits in any form have been or will be received" by any authors. The *Journal* has failed to respond to a request to publish evidence of this conflict.

Privatization of the National Cancer Program

In 1998, ACS created and funded the National Dialogue on Cancer (NDC), cochaired by former President George Bush and Barbara Bush. Included were a wide range of cancer survivor groups, some one hundred representatives of the cancer drug industry, and Shandwick International PR, whose major clients include RJ Reynolds Tobacco Holdings.

Without informing NDC's participants and behind closed doors, ACS then spun off a small legislative committee. Its explicit objective was to advise Congress on the need to replace the 1971 National Cancer Act with a new National Cancer Control Act, which would shift major control of cancer policy from the NCI to the ACS. The proposed Act would also increase NCI funding from this year's $4.6 billion to $14 billion by 2007. The ACS was assisted by Shandwick in drafting the new Act besides managing the NDC.

However, with the February 2002 appointment of ACS President-Elect von Eschenbach as NCI director, the National Cancer Program has been effectively privatized. As a condition of his appointment, von Eschenbach obtained President Bush's agreement to continue as vice chairman of NDC's board of directors, a position he has held since 1998 as a key founder of the dialogue.

Subsequent to von Eschenbach's appointment, NDC was spun off into a nonprofit organization. NDC then hired Edelman, another tobacco PR firm, following a pledge that it would sever its relations with the industry. Edelman represents the Brown & Williamson Tobacco Company and the Altria Group, the parent company of Philip Morris, the nation's biggest cigarette maker; Edelman also represents Kraft and other fast-food and beverage companies now targeted by antiobesity litigation. Edelman is also a board member of the Centers for Disease Control and Prevention Foundation, which fosters relations between the centers, ACS, and the NCI. Edelman has thus become firmly embedded in national cancer policy making. In July 2003, it was discovered that Edelman had reneged on its pledge and was continuing to fight tobacco control programs from its overseas offices. Attempting damage control, Edelman claimed that this was just an oversight. Once more, it agreed to terminate tobacco support programs and to donate this income to charity.

Equally disturbing was the growing secretive collaboration between the NCI and the ACS-NDC complex as revealed in the August 2003 *Cancer Letter*. The latest example was the planned privatization of cancer drug clinical trials together with the creation of a massive tumor tissue bank. This would have cost between $500 million and $1.2 billion to operate apart from construction costs in the billions. This initiative would be privatized, rife with conflicts of interest, exempt from the provisions of the Federal Advisory Committee and Freedom of Information Acts and free from federal technology transfer regulations.

The Cancer Drug Industry 1998 "March" Seriously Misleads the Nation

In September 1998, the cancer drug industry held a national march, led by Gen. Norman Schwarzkopf, under a banner promising Research Cures Cancer. Well-meaning but misled citizens marched for a seemingly important crusade, which, in reality, promoted enormous profits for the drug industry.

Funded with over $3 million by multibillion-dollar cancer drug and with support from mainstream cancer survivor groups, the ACS and, behind the scenes, the NCI stated that the goal of the march was to mobilize grassroots backing for doubling NCI's 1998 budget from $2.6 billion to over $5 billion by 2003.

Some $25 billion and 25 years after President Nixon declared the War against Cancer in 1971, there had been little, if any, significant improvement in treatment and survival rates for most common cancers despite contrary misleading hype by the cancer establishment and periodic claims for the latest miracle cancer drugs, claims that rarely have been substantiated. Meanwhile, the incidence of cancer, particularly nonsmoking cancers, had escalated to epidemic proportions with lifetime cancer risks approaching one in two.

The reason for losing the war against cancer is not a shortage of funds but their gross misallocation. The NCI remains myopically fixated on damage control—diagnosis and treatment—and basic genetic research with indifference to cancer prevention. They have trivialized escalating cancer rates and explained them away as due to faulty lifestyle, to the virtual exclusion of the major role of unwitting and avoidable exposures to industrial carcinogens in air, water, consumer products, and the workplace. The NCI has devoted the most minimal resources and priorities to research on such avoidable causes of cancer, failed to warn the public of these avoidable risks, and failed to provide Congress and regulatory agencies with available scientific information that would allow development of corrective legislative and regulatory action. Responding to recent criticisms, NCI has defensively claimed $1 billion expenditures for cancer prevention. However, more realistic estimates are less than 3% of its total budget.

NCI policies are strongly influenced by pervasive interlocking relationships and conflicts of interest with the cancer drug industry. With taxpayers' money, NCI funded the R & D for the anticancer drug Taxol manufactured by Bristol-Myers. Following completion of expensive clinical trials, the public paid further for developing the drug's manufacturing process. Once completed, NCI gave this industry exclusive right to sell Taxol at an inflationary price, about $5 per milligram, over twenty times the cost of production.

Taxol is not an isolated example. Taxpayers have funded NCI's R & D for over two-thirds of all cancer drugs now on the market. In a surprisingly frank admission, Samuel Broder, NCI director from 1989 to 1995, stated the obvious: "The NCI has become what amounts to a government pharmaceutical company." It should further be noted that the United States spends about five times more on chemotherapy per patient than Great Britain although this is not matched by any difference in survival rates.

Not surprisingly, the NCI has effectively blocked funding for research and clinical trials on promising nontoxic alternative cancer therapies in favor of highly toxic and largely ineffective patented drugs developed by the cancer drug industry.

Rather than increasing NCI's budget, it should be frozen and held hostage to urgent needs for drastic monitored reforms directed to major emphasis on cancer prevention rather than damage control. Furthermore, Congress should subject the NCI drug industry complex to detailed investigation and ongoing scrutiny.

The National Academy of Sciences Challenges the "Special Status" of NCI

A July 29, 2003, National Academy of Sciences (NAS) report on the National Institutes of Health (NIH) was the subject of October 2 bicameral hearings by the House Energy and Commerce and Senate Health, Education, Labor, and Pensions Committees.

The NAS study, requested by Congress, stressed the need to reexamine the "special status granted the National Cancer Institute (NCI) by the 1971

National Cancer Act"; this legislation was responsive to a heavily promoted PR campaign by NCI and American Cancer Society (ACS) representatives. The Act authorized the president to appoint the NCI director and to control its budget, thus bypassing the authority of the overall director of all other twenty-six National Institutes of Health (NIH) and centers. As a result of this anomaly, NCI's $4.6 billion budget, 17% of the NIH, was and remains beyond control of NIH's director.

The NAS expressed further concerns that NCI's special status could cause "an unnecessary rift between [its] goals and mission, and the leadership of NIH." As seriously, NCI's independence has led to its virtual isolation from the public health and general scientific communities.

Beyond the broad scope of the 2003 NAS study and the focus of its Cancer Policy Board on quality health care, NCI's special status has resulted in more serious and generally unrecognized problems. These are largely responsible for losing the war against cancer and include as follows:

- Contrary to NCI's exaggerated claims and misleading public assurances, overall cancer incidence rates and those of childhood and a wide range of nonsmoking adult cancers have escalated over recent decades. Meanwhile, overall mortality rates have remained unchanged and high.
- The leadership of NCI, and its major centers, is marred by pervasive conflicts of interest and a revolving door with industry, particularly the cancer drug industry.
- NCI policies and priorities are imbalanced. They are fixated on damage control—screening, diagnosis, chemoprevention (secondary prevention), treatment, and related research—with minimal priorities for prevention.
- Contrary to requirements of the 1971 Act, the NCI has failed to inform the public of a wide range of avoidable causes of cancer. This denial of the public's right to know has even extended to the suppression of information.
- Since 1998, and in close collaboration with the American Cancer Society (ACS), the National Cancer Program is being surreptitiously privatized.

Prostate Cancer Hope Supplement (PC-Spes)

Breaking news in 2004 reinforced concerns on long-standing major conflicts of interest in the NCI. However, the key role of these conflicts in losing the winnable cancer war remains virtually unrecognized.

Over twenty personal injury suits, filed in LA County Superior Court, allege that the Prostate Cancer Foundation, established in 1995 by Michael Milken, the securities felon turned philanthropist, together with former NCI Director Richard Klausner, and prominent NCI-funded clinicians and researchers have systematically promoted a dangerous dietary supplement.

The supplement, named PC-Spes (PC for *prostate cancer* and Spes, Latin for *hope*), was manufactured and marketed by International Medical Research (IMR) in California. PC-Spes is illegally laced with prescription drugs, including diethylstilbestrol.

PC-Spes has been widely sold to prostate cancer patients and to healthy men to maintain "good prostate health without any adverse reaction." Apart from no evidence for any benefits, several consumers have died, and symptoms and prostate-specific antigen (PSA) levels in cancer patients have been dangerously masked by the supplement's potent estrogenic effects.

NCI's nationwide Comprehensive Cancer Centers also played a major role in promoting the supplement. These include New York's Memorial Sloan-Kettering (MSK), currently headed by former National Institutes of Health (NIH) Director Harold Varmus, and the University of California at Los Angeles and San Francisco. Prominent scientists and oncologists at these centers had conducted clinical trials with the supplement and held shares and controlling interests in IMR, whose directors include Klausner, as executive director of the Gates Foundation Global Health Program. Klausner was then under congressional investigation for violating ethics rules by accepting lecture awards from cancer centers while he was NCI director. Apart from violations of informed consent regulations for patients in clinical trials, the institutions and scientists involved are in violation of California's Corporate Criminal Liability Act, which requires reporting of "any serious concealed danger" as posed by prescription drugs in the supplement.

The PC-Spes revelation illustrates major and long-standing conflicts of interest embedded in the NCI. Following passage of the 1971 National Cancer Act, inaugurating the War against Cancer, President Nixon appointed a three-member NCI executive cancer panel. Benno Schmidt, its first chairman, was a senior drug company executive with close ties to chemical, oil, and steel industries. He was followed in the 1980s by Armand Hammer, the late oil magnate and chairman of Occidental Petroleum, a major manufacturer of industrial chemicals involved in the Love Canal disaster. Not surprisingly, Schmidt and Hammer ignored cancer prevention, let alone the major role of industrial carcinogens. Instead, they focused on the highly profitable development and marketing of cancer drugs. This fox guarding the chicken coop relationship was mirrored in the MSK's Board of Overseers, most of whom were chief executives of drug, petrochemical, and steel industries. This relationship was admitted by Samuel Broder, former NCI director, in a 1998 *Washington Post* interview: "The NCI has become what amounts to a government pharmaceutical company."

NCI's conflicts of interest have still remained unchanged despite the escalating incidence over the last four decades of childhood cancers and adult cancers unrelated to smoking and despite substantial evidence relating these cancers to avoidable exposures to industrial carcinogens.

These conflicts were illustrated in a highly publicized June 30, 2003, CNBC TV program *Titans* (of Cancer Research) *with Maria Bartiromo.* Four cancer titans ignored concerns on cancer prevention while enthusing on claimed major breakthroughs in treatment, particularly with targeted biotech drugs. Included was Varmus, president of MSK Cancer Center and past recipient of major NCI research funds. In 1995, Varmus struck NIH's reasonable pricing clause, protecting against gross industry profiteering from the majority of drugs developed with taxpayer dollars, while giving NIH staff free license to consult with the drug industry. Another titan was Dr. John Mendelsohn, president of NCI's University of Texas MD Anderson Cancer Center, embroiled in conflicts of interest over ImClone's targeted drug Erbitux besides having served as Enron's consultant and board member. Mendelsohn has also been a key player in the National Dialogue on Cancer (NDC), established by the American Cancer Society (ACS) in 1998. The chairman of NDC, recently renamed C-Change, is the urologist Andrew von Eschenbach, prior ACS president-elect and NCI's current director. Of particular interest was the concordance between the NDC and Milken's Prostate Cancer Foundation. As noted in the Washington insider *Cancer Letter*, Milken "is the single most influential player in oncopolitics within the last decade."

NDC's still largely unrecognized objective is the transfer of legislative control of the nation's cancer agenda from the public to the private sector. Straining credulity, NDC's initiative is being handled by Edelman PR, the major international lobbyist for the tobacco industry and fast-food and beverage companies, now targeted by antiobesity litigation.

While the ACS has long been recognized as the tail that wags the NCI dog, this latest example of this relationship was exemplified by the joint planning of a privatized massive tumor tissue bank. This would cost up to $1.2 billion to operate, apart from billions in construction costs. Furthermore, this initiative would be rife with conflicts of interest, exempt from the provisions of the Federal Advisory Committee and Freedom of Information Acts and free from federal technology transfer regulations.

NCI Director Varmus Is Unqualified to Lead the War against Cancer

In October 2010, Senator Chuck Grassley, ranking member of the Senate Finance Committee, wrote to Dr. Harold Varmus, who was appointed director of the National Cancer Institute (NCI). The senator raised questions on the amount of sponsored travel, sometimes a dozen or more trips a year and almost exclusively to international conferences paid for by outside organizations or companies, taken in recent years by "numerous NCI employees, notably senior leadership."

According to *ScienceInsider*, many of the sixteen scientists involved took at least ten trips a year in 2008, 2009, and 2010. However, a subsequent letter from Dr. Varmus and the NIH director, Dr. Francis Collins, claimed that all these travels were part of their scientific work.

Varmus, the current director of the NCI, has a distinguished track record on basic research on cancer treatment. However, this is paralleled by dangerous unawareness of long-standing, well-documented scientific evidence on the causes and prevention of cancer.

As long ago as 1998, Varmus astoundingly claimed, "You can't do experiments to see what causes cancer—it's not an accessible problem, and not the sort of thing scientists can afford to do—everything you do can't be risky." This claim by Varmus that "you can't do research to see what causes cancer" is bizarre, if not absurd.

The International Agency for Research on Cancer (IARC) has published annual reports on carcinogens, largely based on carcinogenicity tests on rodents, since 1964. The National Toxicology Program (NTP) has also published, and continues to do so, systematic and comprehensive reviews on carcinogens, again largely based on carcinogenicity tests, since 1980. Both the IARC and NTP reports detail decades-old unarguable scientific evidence on what causes cancer.

The ignorance or indifference of Varmus to cancer prevention is reinforced by his unrecognized personal conflicts of interest. In 1995, Varmus, then director of the National Institutes of Health, struck the reasonable pricing clause, which protected against exorbitant industry profiteering from the sale of drugs developed with taxpayers' money.

Varmus also gave senior NCI staff free license to consult with the cancer drug industry, a flagrant institutional conflict of interest. In this connection, the 2008 edition of Charity Rating Guide and Watchdog Report listed Varmus with a compensation package of about $2.7 million. According to the *Chronicle of Philanthropy*, this is the highest compensation of directors in over five hundred major nonprofit organizations ever monitored.

As disturbing is the long-standing abdication of responsibility by the NCI, the primary federal institute explicitly charged by President Richard Nixon in 1971 to fight the war against cancer. This charge clearly prioritized the allocation of adequate resources to investigate and eliminate known avoidable causes of cancer. However, while the NCI budget has escalated 25-fold—from $200,000 in 1971 to over $5 billion currently—paradoxically this has been paralleled by an escalation in the incidence of a wide range of cancers. These include liver, 165%; thyroid, 145%; non-Hodgkin's lymphoma, 82%; childhood, 24%; and breast, 19%. These increases also reflect the NCI's long-standing and reckless indifference to prevention, matched by exclusionary emphasis on treatment and related research.

Reflecting these concerns, a July 29, 2003, report by the National Academy of Sciences, requested by Congress, charged that

- the leadership of NCI is marred by pervasive conflicts of interest and a revolving door with industry, particularly the cancer drug industry;
- contrary to NCI's exaggerated claims and misleading public assurances, overall cancer incidence rates, including those of childhood and nonsmoking adults, have sharply escalated over recent decades;
- NCI policies and priorities remain fixated on damage control—screening, diagnosis, and treatment and related research—with minimal priorities for prevention;
- contrary to the requirements of the 1971 Act, the NCI has still failed to inform the public of a wide range of avoidable causes of cancer. This denial of the public's right to know has even been extended to the withholding of readily available scientific information.

These criticisms of the NCI are as germane and timely today as they were seven years ago. However, and disturbingly so, they remain unrecognized by Congress, let alone the public.

The NCI and ACS 2011 Report to the Nation

On March 31, the National Cancer Institute (NCI) and American Cancer Society (ACS) released the related "Annual Report to the Nation on the Status of Cancer, 1975-2007."

The report states that the "overall rates of new cancer diagnosis for men and women combined between 2003 and 2007 combined decreased by an average of slightly less than 1 percent for the same period." However, the report provides no information on incidence rates since 2007 although these are readily available. Moreover, the report admits that "major challenges remain including increasing incidence rates—and that childhood cancer incidence rates continued to increase."

The report quotes a statement by NCI director Dr. Harold Varmus that this decline in incidence rates is "the result of improved methods for preventing several types of cancer." The report also quotes a statement by ACS chief executive officer Dr. John Seffrin that "as we work towards reducing the cancer burden in the population as a whole, it is important that we apply what we know about prevention."

REFORM OF THE NATIONAL CANCER INSTITUTE'S POLICIES IS TWO DECADES OVERDUE[*]

The following reforms were proposed at a February 4, 1992, Washington, D.C., press conference by the Cancer Prevention Coalition, a group of sixty-eight leading cancer prevention and public health experts, past directors of federal agencies, and citizen activists nationwide (appendix A).

1. The National Cancer Institute (NCI) should urgently accord similar emphasis to primary prevention, in terms of budgetary and personnel resources, as all its other programs combined, including screening, diagnosis, treatment and basic research. This major shift in direction should be initiated in the very near future and urgently phased into completion. This shift will require careful monitoring and oversight to prevent misleading retention of old unrelated programs, particularly secondary prevention, under new guises of primary prevention.
2. A high priority for the primary cancer prevention program should be a large scale and ongoing national campaign to inform and educate citizens, the media, regulatory agencies, Congress, the Presidency,

---

[*] Based in part on "THE STOP CANCER BEFORE IT STARTS CAMPAIGN: How to Win the Losing War against Cancer" (Cancer Prevention Coalition Report, 2003). This report was sponsored by eight leading cancer prevention experts and endorsed by over one hundred activists and citizen groups and is based in part on a prior publication in the International Journal of Health Services (see appendix A).

and a wide range of involved industries, that much cancer is avoidable and due to past exposures to chemical and physical carcinogens in air, water, food and the workplace, besides lifestyle factors, particularly smoking. It should, however, be noted that a wide range of occupational exposures and urban air pollution have also been incriminated as causes of lung cancer. Accordingly, the educational campaign should stress the critical importance of identifying and preventing carcinogenic exposures and eliminating or reducing them to the very lowest levels attainable within the earliest practically possible time.

3. The NCI should develop systematic programs for the qualitative and quantitative characterization of carcinogens in air, water, food and the workplace, with particular emphasis on those that are avoidable. Such information should be made available to the general public, and particularly to sub-populations at high risk, by an explicit and ongoing "right-to-know" educational campaign, such as the specific labeling of food and other consumer products with the identity and levels of all carcinogenic ingredients or contaminants. While taking a lead in this program, the NCI should work cooperatively with federal and state regulatory and health agencies and authorities, industry, public health and other professional societies, labor, and community-based citizen groups.

4. The NCI should cooperate with the National Institute of Occupational Safety and Health, and other National Institutes of Health, in investigating and publicizing other chronic toxic effects induced by carcinogens, including reproductive, neurological, hematological and immunological diseases, besides cancer.

5. The NCI should cooperate with the National Institute of Occupational Safety and Health, and other federal institutions including the Centers for Disease Control, to develop large scale programs for monitoring, surveillance and warning of occupational, ethnic, and other sub-population groups at high risk of cancer due to known past exposures to chemical or physical carcinogens.

6. In close cooperation with key regulatory agencies and industry, the NCI should initiate large-scale research programs to develop non-carcinogenic products and processes, as alternatives to those currently based on chemical and physical carcinogens. This program should also include research on the development of economic incentives for the reduction or phase-out of the use of industrial carcinogens, coupled with economic disincentives for their continued use, especially when appropriate non-carcinogenic alternatives are available.

7. The NCI should provide scientific expertise to Congress, federal and state regulatory and health agencies and authorities, and industry on the fundamental scientific principles of carcinogenesis including: the validity of extrapolation to humans of data from valid animal carcinogenicity tests; the invalidity of using insensitive or otherwise questionable epidemiological data to negate the significance of valid animal carcinogenicity tests; and the scientific invalidity of efforts to set "safe levels" or "thresholds" for exposure to individual chemical and physical carcinogens. The NCI should stress that the key to cancer prevention is reducing or avoiding exposure to carcinogens, rather than accepting and attempting to "manage" such risks. Current administration policies are, however, based on highly questionable mathematical procedures of quantitative risk assessment applied to exposures to individual carcinogens, while concomitant exposures to other carcinogens in air, water, food and the workplace are ignored or discounted.

8. The NCI should provide Congress and regulatory agencies with scientific expertise necessary for the development 47 of legislation and regulation of carcinogens. Illustrative of such need is the administration's revocation in 1988 of the 1958 Delaney amendment to the Federal Food Drug and Cosmetic Act, banning the deliberate addition to foods of any level of carcinogen. This critical law was revoked in spite of the overwhelming endorsement of its scientific validity by a succession of expert committees over the past three decades. Disturbingly, the NCI has failed to provide scientific evidence challenging the validity of this revocation, including its likely impact on future cancer rates.

9. The limited programs on routine carcinogenicity testing, now under the authority of the NTP, should be expanded and expedited with the more active and direct involvement of the NCI. (On a cautionary note, it should be emphasized that this program, which is clearly the direct responsibility of the NCI, was transferred to the NTP in 1978 because of mismanagement and disinterest of the NCI). Under-utilized federal resources, particularly national laboratories, should also be involved in carcinogenicity testing programs. The cost of carcinogenicity testing of profitable, and potentially profitable, chemicals should be borne by the industries concerned, and not by the Federal NTP, and ultimately the taxpayer; however, NTP should maintain exclusive responsibility for the testing and reporting of results.

10. The NCI should undertake large scale intramural and extramural research programs to characterize known carcinogenic exposures, both

industrial and lifestyle, for phase-out and elimination within defined early periods.

11. The NCI should substantially expand its intramural and extramural programs on epidemiology research, and develop large-scale programs on sensitive human monitoring techniques, including genetic and, quantitative chemical analysis of body burdens of carcinogens, and focus them specifically on cancer cause and prevention. The NCI should also take a key role in the design, conduct and interpretation of epidemiological investigations of cancer by federal and state regulatory and health agencies and authorities.

12. The NCI should develop large-scale training programs for young scientists in all areas relating to cancer cause and prevention.

13. Continued funding by the NCI of its Comprehensive Cancer Centers should be made contingent on their developing strong community out-reach programs on cancer cause and prevention, as opposed to their present and almost exclusive preoccupation with diagnosis and treatment. Centers should also establish tumor registries focused on identifying environmental and occupational carcinogens, and on the surveillance of occupational and other populations at high risk of cancer.

14. With Congressional oversight and advice from the NIH Office of Scientific Integrity, the NCI should take early action to disclose information on any interlocking financial interests between its Presidential Panel, Advisory Board, advisory committees and others in the cancer establishment, and major pharmaceutical companies involved in cancer drugs and therapy, and other industries. The NCI should also take the necessary precautions to prevent such future conflicts.

15. The three member National Cancer Advisory Panel should be replaced by an executive committee recruited from advisory committees, conforming to standard requirements of the Federal Advisory Committee Act for openness and balanced representation. Half of all appointees to NCI advisory committees should be recruited from scientists with credentials and record of active involvement in cancer cause and prevention. Appointments should also be extended to representatives of citizens', ethnic and women's groups concerned with cancer prevention.

The 1992 statement, however, concluded, "There is no conceivable likelihood that such reforms will be implemented without legislative action . . . Compliance of the NCI should then be assured by detailed and ongoing Congressional oversight and, most critically, by House and Senate Appropriation committees. However, only strong support by the independent scientific and public health communities, together with concerned grassroots citizen groups, will convince Congress and Presidential candidates of the critical and immediate need for such drastic action."

NCI PRESS RELEASES AND HUFFINGTON POST BLOGS

December 12, 1991	Have We Lost the War on Cancer?
December 23, 1991	Losing the Cancer War
June 24, 1993	America Losing Winnable War against Cancer: Experts Urge Clinton to Chart New Course
June 9, 1994	The Cancer Prevention Coalition Calls for the Replacement of the National Cancer Institute Chief
January 25, 1995	Cancer Research Campaign Misleads Public and Congress
August 30, 1996	Cancer War Is Threatened by Recommendations of Presidential Commission
December 18, 1996	We Are Losing the Winnable War against Cancer
April 1, 1998	Cancer "Report Card" Gets a Failing Grade
May 9, 2002	Escalating Incidence of Childhood Cancer Is Ignored by the National Cancer Institute and American Cancer Society
February 20, 2003	U.S. Losing War on Cancer, Ignoring Prevention
February 25, 2003	National Cancer Institute Leadership Is out of Touch with Reality
March 27, 2003	Environmental Causes of Cancer Neglected
November 4, 2003	An Ounce of Prevention
February 23, 2004	Spinning the Losing Cancer War
April 27, 2005	Cancer War Should Focus on Prevention
April 2, 2007	The United Nations Takes the Initiative in the War against Cancer
December 2, 2008	The Obama Cancer Plan
January 23, 2009	The Obama Cancer Plan Must Prioritize Prevention

December 12, 1991

Chicago Tribune

HAVE WE LOST THE WAR ON CANCER?

As America debates the health-care crisis, the time has come to look more closely at the biggest ticket item, cancer. Huge expenditures on cancer only make sense if we are making progress. In fact, we are moving backwards.

A recent report from the American Hospital Association states the facts. Per-case Medicare payments for cancer now exceed those for any other disease, and are rising more rapidly than for any other disease. By the year 2000, the report chillingly predicts cancer will become the leading cause of death and "dominant specialty" of American medicine.

There are no accurate figures on cancer's overall cost. The best estimate is more than $100 billion a year. Where does it all go?

The direct costs of cancer include more than 50 million visits to physicians, a million operations, at least 750,000 radiation treatment and uncountable diagnostic tests. Many highly profitable magnetic resonance imaging facilities are owned by the doctors who prescribe the tests, a situation the editor of the New England Journal of Medicine called "a terrible conflict of interest."

Indirect costs of cancer include research and the loss of income from premature disability or death. Nearly $20 billion has been given—virtually without strings—to the National Cancer Institute since 1971. The American Cancer Society solicits more than $330 million a year from the public. The budget of the Memorial Sloan-Kettering Cancer Center in New York is more than $350 million.

Few could begrudge the cancer establishment these huge costs if they resulted in significant progress. However, the incidence of cancer has escalated to epidemic levels. Since 1950, adjusting for the aging population, incidence rates have increased by 40 percent. Rates for cancers of the breast, prostate, and colon in males have increased by 60 percent, childhood cancers by 30 percent, and other less common cancers by over 100 percent. Cancer now strikes one in three and kills one in four, with half a million deaths last year.

Contrary to the optimistic and misleading hype of the National Cancer Institute, American Cancer Society, Sloan-Kettering and other cancer centers, our ability to treat and cure cancer has not materially improved over decades. Apart from rare cancers, five-year survival rates for common advanced cancers have scarcely improved. For example, the mortality rate for non-localized breast cancer has remained a static 18 percent over the last 40 years.

Meanwhile, treatment has become highly toxic, sophisticated and expensive and a major source of profit to giant pharmaceutical companies closely interlocked with the cancer establishment. Bone marrow transplantation comes with a very high price tag—about $100,000 per patient—and a very low chance of success. Other modern treatments, such as interferon, interluekin-2 and gene therapy, are so toxic that other drugs have to be developed and used in efforts to counteract their side effects.

Prevention is the key to reducing the inflationary impact of cancer. Our total environment had become progressively permeated with industrial carcinogens in air, food, water and the workplace. The 1958 Delaney law, which banned the deliberate introduction of any level of carcinogenic pesticides and other chemicals into our food supply, has been recently gutted in favor of an allegedly "negligible risk" standard by the Bush administration, supported by a rollover Congress. Not a word of support for the Delaney law, the scientific validity of which has been repeatedly endorsed by independent expert committees, has come from the National Cancer Institute and American Cancer Society. This cancer establishment has also remained silent while the administration rolls back regulations on dioxin and asbestos and refuses to phase out the manufacture and use of industrial carcinogens, contributing still further to the future toll of avoidable cancer.

Besides prevention, there is a critical need to mount an intensive and fair-minded investigation of promising non-toxic innovative cancer therapies. Many such therapies are both low-cost and non-patentable. Last year, the congressional Office of Technology Assessment reported on some 200 papers supporting such innovative therapies and recommended that the cancer institute actively investigate them. It refused.

Twenty years ago this month, responding to pressures from the cancer establishment and promises to cure cancer by the Bicentennial, President Nixon signed the National Cancer Act and inaugurated the "War Against Cancer." The war is now all but lost, and this realty must be forced on the National Cancer Institute and the American Cancer Society by Congress and the public. However, only a grass-roots movement of activist citizens will convince politicians and presidential candidates of the need for drastic action.

ENDORSER:

Ralph Moss
Author, *The Cancer Industry*

December 23, 1991

USA Today

LOSING THE CANCER WAR

On Dec. 23, 1971, President Nixon signed the National Cancer Act. The "War Against Cancer" was inaugurated, and the cure for cancer was promised by the Bicentennial.

Twenty years, billions of dollars and millions of deaths later, no cure is in sight. We're losing the war.

Cancer now strikes one in three and kills one in four Americans—500,000 last year alone. Since 1950, overall incidence rates have increased by 40%. Cancers of the breast, of prostate and colon in men have escalated 60%; cancers in children, 30%. Less common cancers have increased more than 100%.

These statistics are frightening but understate the full story. Cancer rates are even higher among blacks, urban poor and 11 million workers in petrochemical, metal and nuclear industries. Over recent decades, our whole environment—food, air, water and workplace—has become progressively permeated with cancer-causing industrial chemicals.

Our ability to cure most advanced cancers scarcely has improved since 1971. For example, the five-year survival rate for non-localized breast cancer remains a static 18%.

But what about emerging "cures" we were promised, such as Taxol or genetic engineering? Remember the cancer vaccine? Remember interferon, miracle cures of the '70s?

In truth, few scientists believe their work will result in cures any time soon. But such hype secures next year's funding for hungry bureaucrats and researchers.

This "cancer establishment" pushes highly toxic and expensive drugs, patented by major pharmaceutical firms which also have close links to cancer centers. Is it any wonder they refuse to investigate innovative approaches developed outside their own institutions?

Last year, the Office of Technology Assessment found almost 200 scientific studies supporting such methods. It urged the National Center Institute to investigate. But NCI continues to stonewall.

The same cancer establishment, with Congress' tacit approval, stands by as the Bush Administration guts the Delaney Amendment, the 1958 law banning deliberate introduction of pesticides and other avoidable carcinogens into our food.

We clearly need a complete restructuring of the losing war against cancer. Prevention must get the highest priority. Industrial carcinogens must be phased out or banned. Innovative non-toxic therapies must get independent evaluation.

Until then, Congress must refuse to fund NCI and the public should boycott the bloated American Cancer Society.

Only such a grass-roots movement of determined citizens can force politicians—including presidential candidates—to make the fight against cancer a top national priority.

ENDORSER:

Ralph Moss
Author, *The Cancer Industry*

June 24, 1993

AMERICA LOSING WINNABLE WAR AGAINST CANCER: EXPERTS URGE CLINTON TO CHART NEW COURSE

The Cancer Prevention Coalition, a national organization of doctors, cancer researchers and public health officials, today released a letter to President Clinton warning that the nation is losing a winnable war against cancer and urging a new federal strategy that emphasizes preventing exposure to cancer-causing substances.

Led by Drs. Samuel Epstein, University of Illinois cancer prevention expert, John Spratt, oncologist and surgeon affiliated with the University of Louisville Medical School, and Peter Orris, Medical Director at Chicago's Mount Sinai Hospital's Occupational Medical Program, 50 leading cancer experts called on the White House "to make prevention the guiding strategy for a successful war on this dread disease."

"Despite significant gains in the treatment of certain cancers, America is still losing the war," declared Dr. Epstein. Citing the government's own statistics, Epstein pointed to the 43% increase between 1950 and 1988 in cancer incidence rates and the failure to improve cancer survival rates as evidence that "not enough is being done to protect citizens from exposure to cancer-causing substances."

"Over the past 20 years," argued Dr. Epstein, "spending has increased nearly 10-fold, yet cancer incidence rates have climbed by more than 16 percent." Furthermore, added Epstein, "5-year survival rates have remained flat at about 50% for men and women and at about 38% for African-Americans."

The Cancer Prevention Coalition called on the President to:

- Place equal budgetary emphasis on cancer cause and prevention alongside research, diagnosis and treatment
- Phase-out the manufacture and use of industrial carcinogens and institute a crash program to develop safer alternatives
- Expand the testing of chemicals and chemical compounds for carcinogenicity

"Pesticide residues, chemicals in the workplace, benzene in gasoline, air and water pollution, and toxic waste dumps pose cancer threats to exposed populations. Since there is no such thing as a 'safe' exposure level, and since many forms of cancer are now clearly associated with exposure to these substances, it is unconscionable that the federal government allocates so few resources to identifying and testing cancer-causing chemicals and preventing public exposure," said Dr. Peter Orris.

"Clearly," said Orris, "our government is not doing enough to protect workers and the public from exposure to chemicals in the workplace and environment that cause or trigger cancer. Much has been done to inform the public about the deathly hazards of smoking. Similar efforts are needed to educate the public about the proliferation of cancer-causing chemicals in our workplaces, in the food we eat, the water we drink and the air breathe," said Orris.

"The National Cancer Institute has failed its mission," argued Dr. John S. Spratt. "The NCI has given first priority to chemotherapy, a treatment of marginal benefit. The NCI needs a new direction. It must focus on preventing the onset of cancer in the first place, given that by the year 2000, cancer will be America's single most expensive disease."

June 24, 1993

LETTER TO PRESIDENT CLINTON

Dear President Clinton:

America is losing a winnable war against a dreaded disease, cancer. We can prevent unnecessary suffering and deaths only by radically reforming federal cancer policy to emphasize prevention rather than just diagnosis, treatment and basic research. The undersigned cancer and public health professionals urge you to undertake a thorough reform of cancer policies throughout your Administration, and make prevention the guiding strategy for the war against cancer.

Over the last decade, some five million Americans died of cancer. Cancer now strikes one in three and kills one in four Americans, with over 500,000 deaths last year. Cancer incidence rates in the white U.S. population (adjusted for increasing longevity) have increased by 43% from 1950-1988. During this time breast cancer has increased by 60%, childhood cancer by 21%, and other cancers by over 100%. A recent report by the American Hospital Association predicts that cancer will become the leading cause of death by the year 2000, and the "dominant specialty of American medicine."

There is substantial evidence that many of these cancers are due to avoidable exposures to industrial carcinogens in air, water, food, and the workplace. Meanwhile, our ability to treat and cure most cancers has remained virtually unchanged. From 1973-1988, 5-year survival rates have remained about 50% for the overall population and only 38% for Afro-Americans. The cancer mortality rate for black males is over four times higher than for white males.

The annual costs of cancer, an estimated $110 billion (nearly 2% of the GNP), are major inflationary factors in the current health care crisis with Per-case Medicare payments exceeding those for any other disease. These costs seriously threaten your Administration's efforts to provide health care to all Americans.

Even as cancer incidence escalates the National Cancer Institute (NCI) continues to mislead the public and Congress with claims that we are "winning" the war against cancer. The NCI which still attributes most cancer to smoking and dietary fat, discounts or ignores the causal role of avoidable exposures to occupational and environmental carcinogens and devotes minimal priorities and resources in its $1.9 billion budget to these concerns.

Your Administration offers great hopes for changing the nation's misdirected cancer policies and reversing the cancer epidemic. We attach a statement of reforms as general guidelines for redefining the mission and priorities of the

NCI. We urgently request a meeting with your staff to discuss how we can work together to win the war against cancer.

Samuel S. Epstein, MD
Professor of Occupational and Environmental Medicine
The Chairman Cancer Prevention Coalition

CO-SIGNATORIES:

Dan Abrahamson, MD, PhD, Professor Public Affairs, University of Minnesota

Nicholas A. Ashford, PhD, JD, Associate Professor Technology and Policy, Massachusetts Institute of Technology, Cambridge

Louis S. Beliczky, MS, MPH, Director Industrial Hygiene Safety, United Rubber Workers, AFL-CIO

Rosalie Bertell, PhD, President International Institute of Public Health Concern, Toronto, Canada

Eula Bingham, PhD, University of Cincinnati Medical Center (former Assistant Secretary of Labor, OSHA)

Irwin D. Bross, PhD, President Metatechnology, Buffalo (former Director Biostatistics Roswell Park Memorial Institute)

Barry Castleman, PhD, Environmental Consultant, Baltimore

David Christiani, MD, Associate Professor Occupational Medicine. Harvard School Public Health

Richard Clapp, PhD, Director John Snow. Institute Boston

Paul Connett, PhD, Professor Chemistry. St. Lawrence University, New York

Brian Dolan, MD, Internist. Santa Monica, California

Michael Ellenbecker, PhD, Professor Work Environment. University Massachusetts Lowell

George Friedman-Jimenez, MD. Medical Director. Occupational and Environmental Health Clinic, Bellevue Hospital, NY

Richard Garcia, PhD, Entomologist. University of California, Berkeley

Jack Geiger, MD, Professor Community Medicine CUNY Medical School, New York

Jay Gould, PhD, Director Radiation and Public Health Project, New York

Stephen Hessl, MD, Chairman Division Medicine. Cook County Hospital, Chicago, Professor Occupational and Environmental Medicine, University Illinois

Thomas Higginbotham, DO, Internist, Colorado Springs

Ruth Hubbard, PhD, Emerita Professor Biology, Harvard University

Howard Kippen, MD, MPH, Professor Environmental and Occupational Health, Robert Wood

Johnson Medical School, Piscataway, New Jersey

Marc Lappe, PhD, Professor Health Policy and Ethics, University Illinois College of Medicine, Chicago

Marvin Legator, PhD, Professor Preventive Medicine and Community Health, University Texas, Galveston

Brian Leibovitz, PhD, Editor-in-Chief. *Journal Optimal Nutrition*. Davis, California

Charles Levenstein, PhD, Professor Work Environment, University Massachusetts, Lowell

Edward A. Lichter, MD, Professor Internal Medicine. University Illinois College of Medicine

William Lijinsky, PhD (former Director Chemical Carcinogenesis, Frederick Cancer Research Center, Maryland)

Thomas Mancuso, MD, Emeritus Professor Occupational Medicine, University Pittsburgh

Franklin E. Mirer, PhD, Director Health and Safety Department United Auto Workers, Detroit

David Monroe, PhD, Toxicologist. Oak Harbor, Washington

Vicente Navarro, MD, PhD, Professor Health Policy, Johns Hopkins University

John W. Olney, MD, Professor Medicine. Washington University School Medicine, St. Louis

Peter Orris, MD, Senior Physician, Division Occupational Medicine, Cook County Hospital

Brandon P. Reines, DVM., President Center Health Science Policy, Washington, D.C.

Knut Ringen, Dr.Ph., Director Center to Protect Workers Rights. Washington, D.C. (former Director Labor's Health and Safety Fund North America, Washington, D.C.)

Kenneth Rosenman, MD, Professor Medicine, Michigan State University, Lansing

DS Sarma, PhD, Department of Pathology, University of Toronto, Canada

Ruth Shearer, PhD, Toxicologist. Issaquah, Washington

Janette D. Sherman, MD, Internist. Alexandria, Virginia

Victor Sidel, MD, Distinguished University Professor Social Medicine. Albert Einstein College Medicine, New York

Joseph H. Skom, MD, Professor Clinical Medical Northwestern University Medical School, Chicago

John Spratt, MD, American Cancer Society. Professor Oncology and Professor Surgery, Brown

Cancer Center. University Louisville Medical School, Kentucky

EJ Sternglass, PhD, Emeritus Professor Radiological Physics. University, Pittsburgh Medical School

Carlo Tamburro, MD, Professor Medicine and Chief Division Occupational Medicine.

Brown Cancer Center, University Louisville Medical School, Kentucky

George Wald, Nobel Laureate, Harvard University

George Washington University, Washington, D.C.

Thomas Woodcock, MD, Professor Medicine and George Wald, Nobel Laureate, Harvard University

Laura Welch, MD, Associate Professor Medicine, Director Division Occupational and Environmental Medicine Head Division Haematology and Oncology, Brown Cancer Center University Louisville Medical School, Kentucky

Charles Wurster, PhD, Associate Professor Environmental Toxicology. Marine Sciences Research Center, SUNY. Stony Brook, New York

Arthur Zahalsky, PhD, Professor Immunology, Department biological Sciences, Southern Illinois University, Edwardsville, Illinois

Grace Ziem, PhD, Consultant Occupational and Environmental Health, Baltimore

June 9, 1994

THE CANCER PREVENTION COALITION CALLS FOR THE REPLACEMENT OF THE NATIONAL CANCER INSTITUTE DIRECTOR

In a letter sent today to President Clinton, the Cancer Prevention Coalition (CPC), a nation-wide coalition of cancer prevention experts, and citizen activists, calls for the immediate replacement of Dr. Samuel Broder, director of the National Cancer Institute (NCI).

According to Dr. Samuel Epstein, Chairman of CPC, "Dr. Broder has recently attempted to distance himself from serious scientific fraud, involving NCI breast cancer treatment trials, coordinated by University of Pittsburgh's Dr. Fisher. However, clear evidence of this fraud, involving taxpayers' dollars, was well known some three years ago to Dr. Broder who failed to take any corrective action, let alone inform cancer patients. Furthermore, NCI has embarked on a breast cancer 'prevention' trial on healthy women treated with Tamoxifen, also coordinated by Dr. Fisher. NCI's prevention claims are scientifically questionable if not reckless, and the patient consent forms misleadingly trivialize serious toxic effects of the drug, including aggressive uterine and liver cancers."

Additionally, the CPC directors charge NCI "with having misled the public and Congress into believing that we are winning the war against cancer. In fact, we are losing this war. Cancer rates are escalating to epidemic proportions, now striking more than one in three and killing more than one in four. Also, our ability to treat and cure most cancers has not improved for decades. Moreover, the inflationary costs of cancer are a major factor in the current health care crisis. Meanwhile, NCI is indifferent if not hostile to cancer prevention."

The letter to the President details the following charges:

- NCI allocates less than 2.5% of its $2 billion annual budget to research on avoidable exposures to environmental and occupational carcinogens.
- NCI has been silent with regard to the contamination of hot dogs with the highly potent carcinogen dimethylnitrosamine, although this has been known since the early 1970's. A recent study links frequent hot dog consumption with childhood leukemia and brain cancer.
- The Institute has failed to warn some fifty million women who use permanent hair dyes of the risks of lymphomas and other cancers.

The Coalition concluded, "Dr. Broder's replacement by a qualified scientist with balanced interest in prevention, treatment and basic research is clearly overdue. But this is not enough. Radical reforms are needed to redirect NCI policies and priorities, with greater emphasis on cancer prevention by research informational, and interventional programs."

January 25, 1995

CANCER RESEARCH CAMPAIGN MISLEADS PUBLIC AND CONGRESS

A statement by national organizations representing over 5 million Americans warned of misleading efforts by treatment groups and the cancer drug industry to allocate more tax dollars towards funding cancer research.

The statement responded to a Washington, D.C. kick-off of the National Coalition for Cancer Research's industry-sponsored "Research Cures Cancer" campaign, which is lobbying Congress to increase support for the National Cancer Institute's (NCI) programs.

The statement sent a message to policymakers that further funding is not going to cure cancer. It stressed that NCI's priorities are fixated on research on treatment and molecular biology, while issues of environmental and workplace-induced cancers are trivialized. The reason for the failed war against cancer is not a shortage of funds but their gross misallocation. NCI has devoted minimal funding to cancer prevention. Furthermore, NCI has failed to inform Congress and the public of a wide range of avoidable causes of environmental and occupational cancers.

The organizations concluded by calling for an appointment of a new director at NCI who is more responsive to growing national concerns on prevention of the cancer epidemic.

Cancer Research Campaign Misleads Public and Congress

On January 25, 1995 in Washington, D.C., the National Coalition for Cancer Research will launch an industry-funded "Research Cures Cancer" campaign which misleads Congress and the public into the groundless belief that further research is the answer to the cancer epidemic. The Coalition, sponsored by the American Cancer Society and the cancer drug industry, is lobbying Congress and taxpayers to provide the National Cancer Institute (NCI) with more research funding.

Twenty-five years since President Nixon and Congress inaugurated the National Cancer Act, the war against cancer has failed. In spite of over $25 billion of taxpayers funding, cancer rates have escalated to epidemic proportions while our ability to treat and cure most cancers remains largely unchanged.

For decades, NCI policy and priorities have remained narrowly fixated on research on treatment and basic molecular biology. Despite its questionable relevance, molecular biology receives over 50% of NCI's $2 billion annual budget. Nevertheless, molecular biologist and current director of the National Institutes of Health, Dr. Harold Varmus, is encouraging still more emphasis on basic molecular biology research in the NCI.

The reason for the failed war against cancer is not a shortage of funds but their gross misallocation. NCI has directed a minimal priority to cancer prevention. Furthermore, NCI has failed to inform Congress and the public of a wide range of avoidable carcinogens in the air, water, food, consumer products and the workplace. Research on such exposures receives a miniscule 5% of NCI's annual budget. Reduction of exposures to carcinogens in the workplace and the environment are likely to reverse the current epidemic.

With the NCI directorship being vacated next month, it is time to see the NCI face up to escalating cancer rates and its imbalanced preoccupation with research on treatment and molecular biology. As organizations representing 5 million Americans, we demand that President Clinton appoint a leading scientist with a strong credentials and clear commitment to cancer prevention as director of the NCI.

The Cancer Prevention Coalition and the co-signing organizations also demand that:

- NCI must be held accountable for its failed policies and the $25 billion in taxpayer support in the war against cancer.
- NCI must undergo radical reforms in its programs, priorities, and leadership.
- Cancer prevention must receive greater emphasis in NCI policies.
- The NCI budget must be held hostage to such reforms under the terms of the Government Performance and Results Act of 1993.

CO-SIGNING ORGANIZATIONS:

Breast Cancer Action
San Francisco, CA

Cancer Prevention Coalition
Chicago, IL

Center for Constitutional Rights
New York, NY

Center for Media and Democracy
Madison, WI

Citizen Action
Washington, DC

Environmental Research Foundation
Annapolis, MD

Food and Water, Inc.
Marshfield, VT

Greenpeace USA
Chicago, IL

Mother Jones Magazine
San Francisco, CA

Pesticide Action Network
San Francisco, CA

Project Impact
Oakland, CA

Pure Food Campaign
Washington, DC

Radiation and Public Health Project
New York, NY

Women's Community Cancer Project
Boston, MA

Women's Environment and Development Organization
New York, NY

August 30, 1996

CANCER WAR IS THREATENED BY RECOMMENDATIONS OF PRESIDENTIAL COMMISSION

Cancer rates will skyrocket, if the June 13, 1996 recommendations of the President's Commission on Risk Assessment are implemented. "These recommendations will open the floodgates to cancer-causing and other toxic industrial chemicals in the air, water, food and the workplace," warned Samuel Epstein, M.D.

The Presidential Commission is proposing to roll back regulation of carcinogenic and other toxic industrial chemicals. It promises to "manage" health risks rather than preventing them. It also discredits animal tests for carcinogens and allows for "safe" exposure levels; the Commission's report goes to the President and Congress in early October. Similar proposals by the Environmental Protection Agency have recently met with widespread consumer and scientific opposition.

Since 1971, when President Nixon and Congress inaugurated the National Cancer Act, the National Cancer Institute's war against cancer has failed. After $30 billion in taxpayer spending, the incidence of cancer has reached epidemic proportions—now striking more than one in three and killing more than one in four—while our ability to treat and cure most cancers remains largely unchanged. Cancer costs are now over $100 billion dollars a year and are a major factor in the current health care crisis; per-case Medicare payments for cancer now exceed those for any other disease. "We are losing the war against cancer and this would be the knock-out punch" concluded Dr. Epstein.

December 18, 1996

WE ARE LOSING THE WINNABLE WAR AGAINST CANCER

Contrary to the recent highly publicized December 1996 claims by the National Cancer Institute (NCI), Americans are getting more cancer than ever before. And rather than getting better, the problem is getting worse.

The claim by the NCI, announced in anticipation of the twenty-fifth Anniversary of the December 23, 1971 National Cancer Act launching "the War against Cancer," asserts that we have "turned the tide against cancer." As evidence, the NCI pointed to a "nearly 3% reduction" in cancer mortality from 1991-95, mostly due to a decline in lung cancer deaths from smoking in men, and to improved access to health care, particularly among African Americans.

Most importantly, while cancer deaths have declined very modestly, the number of people *getting* cancer in America has been and still is on the rise. The "tide against cancer" incidence has not only *not* been turned back, but continues to escalate now striking more than one in three, up from an incidence of one in four a few decades ago. In fact, cancer incidence is still increasing overall and for a broad range of cancers at all ages, including: childhood leukemia and brain cancer; testicular cancer, non-Hodgkin's lymphoma and melanoma among young and middle age adults; and prostate and breast cancers in older groups. Cancer incidence—the total number of people getting cancer as opposed to the smaller numbers developing fatal cancers—is a much more significant and accurate measure of cancer trends than is mortality.

Further, the picture on mortality, when examined closely, is less rosy than the NCI would have us believe. Since 1991, cancer mortality rates for Americans over the age of 65 continues its four-decade old climb, even after statistical adjustments for an aging population. Also, there has been a sharp increase in mortality from non-smoking related cancers, including multiple myeloma, non-Hodgkin's lymphoma, chronic leukemia, and pancreatic cancer.

Smoking apart, NCI's latest announcement makes only minimal reference to cancer prevention. More specifically, NCI continues to ignore or trivialize the wealth of information on avoidable exposures to petrochemical and other carcinogens in the workplace, air, water food, cosmetics, and other consumer products and on the substantial scientific evidence linking such undisclosed exposures to the cancer epidemic. This clearly reflects the continuing fixation of the NCI, and also the American Cancer Society, on diagnosis, treatment and basic molecular biology research with minimal priority for cancer prevention; cancer prevention programs receive only some 2% of NCI's $2.2 billion annual budget.

"Rather than optimistic and ill-based assurances, the latest in a long series of smoke and mirror "breakthroughs" since 1971, drastic reforms shifting NCI priorities to cancer prevention are key to winning the losing war against cancer," urges Samuel S. Epstein, M.D, Chairman of the Cancer Prevention Coalition and Professor of Occupational and Environmental Medicine at the School of Public Health, University of Illinois Medical Center, Chicago. Such critical reforms are unlikely unless the public can be mobilized, along an AIDS Act-Up grass-roots model, to act on the belated realization that the cancer war is too important to be trusted to its myopic generals and big government bureaucrats.

April 1, 1998

CANCER "REPORT CARD" GETS A FAILING GRADE

At a highly publicized March 12, 1998, Washington, DC press briefing, the National Cancer Institute (NCI) and American Cancer Society (the cancer establishment), together with the Centers for Disease Control and Prevention, released a "Report Card" announcing the recent reversal of "an almost 20-year trend of increasing cancer cases and death," as detailed in the March 15 issue of the journal *Cancer*. "These numbers are the first proof that we are on the right track," enthused NCI director Dr. Richard Klausner. This news received extensive and uncritical nation-wide media coverage.

These claims were based on a comparison between NCI's published statistics for 1973-1990 and 1973-1995. However, the more recent information remains unpublished and, according to senior NCI statistician Dr. Lynn Ries, is still being analyzed. More importantly, a critical review of the *Cancer* publication is hardly reassuring. The claimed reversal in overall mortality rates is not only minimal but exaggerated. It is largely due to a reduction in lung cancer deaths from smoking in men, reflecting personal lifestyle choices, and to improved access to health care rather than to any improvements in treatment and survival rates. Additionally, any true decline would be considerably less if the mortality rates were appropriately based on the current age distribution of the U.S. population, rather than that of 1970, with its relatively higher representation of younger age groups, as misleadingly calculated by NCI. These criticisms are in general consistent with those detailed in a May 1997 *New England Journal of Medicine* article, "Cancer Undefeated," by former NCI epidemiologist Dr. John Bailar.

The claimed reversal in the incidence of cancers of "all sites" is minimal and statistically insignificant, as are similar claims for leukemia and prostate cancer. Even this minimal reduction of prostate cancer is highly questionable as admitted by Report Card authors: "The decreased incidence rates [of prostate cancer] may be the result of decreased utilization of PSA [prostate specific antigen] screening tests . . . during the early 1990's." While there were significant reductions in the incidence of lung, colon/rectum and bladder cancers, there were significant and sharp increases in uterine cancer, melanoma, and non-Hodgkin's lymphoma. Moreover, there was no decline in breast cancer rates, which remain unchanged at their current high level. Curiously, no reference at all was made to testicular cancer in young adults nor to childhood cancer, whose rates have dramatically increased in recent decades.

The Report Card apart, there are disturbing questions on the reliability of NCI's incidence statistics. This is well illustrated by wild reported variations since 1973 for the percent changes in the incidence of childhood cancer:

1973-1980	+21%
1973-1989	+10%
1973-1990	+1%
1973-1991	-8%
1973-1994	+31%

The Report Card's optimistic and misleading assurances, the latest in a series of smoke and mirror break-through since 1971 when President Nixon launched the "War Against Cancer," are designed to divert attention from the escalating incidence of cancer, which has reached epidemic proportions. Cancer now strikes 1 in 2 men and 1 in 3 women, up from an incidence of 1 in 4 a few decades ago. Meanwhile, our ability to treat and cure most cancer, apart from relatively infrequent cancers particularly those of children, remains virtually unchanged. The Report Card is also designed to neutralize criticism of NCI's intransigent fixation on diagnosis, treatment, and basic genetic research, coupled with indifference to prevention, which receives minimal priorities and resources—less than 5% of NCI's budget. Further illustrative is the fact that NCI has never testified before Congress or regulatory agencies on the substantial published evidence on the wide range of carcinogenic industrial contaminants of air, water, the workplace, and consumer products—food, household products, and cosmetics—and on the need to prevent such avoidable and involuntary exposures. Nor has NCI recognized the public's right-to-know of such critical information, which plays a major role in escalating cancer rates, nor have they developed community outreach prevention programs. Finally, the Report Card is designed to further buttress aggressive lobbying by the cancer establishment and cancer drug industry for a major increase in NCI's budget from the current $2.6 billion, up from $223 million in 1971, to the requested $3.2 billion in 1999.

Rather than increasing NCI's bloated budget, drastic reforms are needed to explicitly re-orient its mission and priorities to cancer causes and prevention.

May 9, 2002

ESCALATING INCIDENCE OF CHILDHOOD CANCER REMAINS IGNORED BY THE NATIONAL CANCER INSTITUTE

Since passage of the 1971 National Cancer Act, the incidence of childhood cancer has steadily escalated to alarming levels. Childhood cancers have increased by 26% overall, while the incidence of particular cancers has increased still more: acute lymphocytic leukemia, 62%; brain cancer, 50%; and bone cancer, 40%. The NCI, besides by the "charitable" American Cancer Society (ACS), have failed to inform the public, let alone Congress and regulatory agencies, of this alarming information. As importantly, they have failed to publicize well-documented scientific information on avoidable causes responsible for the increased incidence of childhood cancer. Examples include:

- Over 20 U.S. and international studies have incriminated paternal and maternal exposures (pre-conception, during conception and post-conception) to a wide range of occupational carcinogens as major causes of childhood cancer.
- There is substantial evidence on the risks of brain cancer and leukemia in children from frequent consumption of nitrite-dyed hot dogs; consumption during pregnancy has been similarly incriminated. Nitrites, added to meat for coloring purposes, have been shown to react with natural chemicals in meat (amines) to form a potent carcinogenic nitrosamine.
- Consumption of non-organic fruits and vegetables, particularly in baby food, contaminated with high concentrations of multiple residues of carcinogenic pesticides, poses major risks of childhood cancer, besides delayed cancers in adult life.
- Numerous studies have shown strong associations between childhood cancers, particularly brain cancer, non-Hodgkin's lymphoma and leukemia, and domestic exposure to pesticides from uses in the home, including pet flea collars, lawn and garden; another major source of exposure is commonplace use in schools.
- Use of lindane, a potent carcinogen in shampoos for treating lice and scabies, infesting about six million children annually, is associated with major risks of brain cancer; lindane is readily absorbed through the skin.
- Treatment of children with Ritalin for "Attention Deficit Disorders" poses risks of cancer, in the absence of informed parental consent.

Ritalin has been shown to induce highly aggressive rare liver cancers in rodents at doses comparable to those prescribed to children.
• Maternal exposure to ionizing radiation, especially in late pregnancy, is strongly associated with excess risks of childhood leukemia.

It is of particular significance that the cancer establishment ignored the continuing increase in the incidence of childhood cancer in its heavily promoted, but highly arguable, March 1998 "claim to have reversed an almost 20-year trend of increasing cancer cases."

The failure of the NCI to warn of these avoidable cancer risks reflects mind-sets fixated on damage control—screening, diagnosis, and treatment—and basic genetic research, with indifference to primary prevention, as defined by research and public education on avoidable causes of cancer.

The minimal priorities for prevention reflects mind-sets and policies and not lack of resources. NCI's annual budget has increased some 20-fold since passage of the 1971 Act, from $220 million to $4.2 billion. NCI expenditures on primary prevention have been estimated as under 4% of its budget.

It should be particularly stressed that fetuses, infants and children are much more vulnerable and sensitive to toxic and carcinogenic exposures than are adults. It should also be recognized that the majority of carcinogens also induce other chronic toxic effects, especially in fetuses, infants and children. These include endocrine disruptive and reproductive, hematological, immunological and genetic, for which there are no available incidence trend data comparable to those for cancer.

The continued silence of the NCI on avoidable causes of childhood, besides a wide range of other, cancers is in flagrant denial of the specific charge of the 1971 National Cancer Act "to disseminate cancer information to the public." As seriously, this silence is a denial of the public's inalienable democratic right-to-know of information directly impacting on their health and lives, and of their right to influence public policy.

ENDORSER:

Quentin D. Young, MD
Chairman of Health and Medicine Policy Research Group
Past President of the American Public Health Association.

February 20, 2003

U.S. LOSING WAR ON CANCER, IGNORING PREVENTION

Leading players in the war on cancer should do more to educate the American public about how to minimize its risk of contracting the disease, according to a February 2003 report from the Cancer Prevention Coalition (CPC).

Americans face increasing cancer risks from occupational and environmental exposure to industrial carcinogens, the report finds, but established government and nonprofit cancer organizations are fixated on treatment rather than prevention.

This report makes it clear that we are losing the war against cancer. But, there are opportunities for reversing this trend.

Based on available data, the overall incidence of cancers in the American population is on the rise. Men have a little less than a one in two lifetime risk of developing cancer, for women the risk is a bit more than one in three.

Adjusted to reflect the aging population, the U.S. cancer incidence is up some 24 percent from 1973 to 1999. Mortality rates are up some 30 percent over the same time period.

But some argue these numbers are misleading, as the medical community's ability to identify cancer has improved over that time period. Still, cancer kills some 550,000 Americans each year and is the second leading cause of death. Some 1.3 million Americans contract cancer each year.

And the American war on cancer has been undermined by the myopic focus on treatment.

The NCI has been silent on a wide range of avoidable causes of cancer, other than personal lifestyle choices such as smoking. However, there is enough evidence to warn people of the presence of industrial pollutants, the concentrations of pesticides in nonorganic fruits and vegetables and the possible risks of irradiated foods.

The NCI has taken no strong stand on the dangers from carcinogenic exposures from pesticides or hazardous industrial waste. This has tacitly encouraged powerful corporate polluters and industries to continue manufacturing carcinogenic products. These organizations tend to "blame the victim" for contracting cancer, he said, rather than explore the environmental causation that could be responsible for their illness.

Clearly the public should have access to a registry compiled by NCI of "avoidable carcinogens," and Congress may need to step in to ensure this happens.

This mandate explicitly comes from the 1971 National Cancer Act, signed by President Richard Nixon, and was strengthened by amendments in 1988 that called for "an expanded and intensified research program for the prevention of cancer caused by occupational or environmental exposure to carcinogens."

The Cancer Prevention Coalition report calls on states to enact the equivalent of a toxics use reduction act passed in 1989 by Massachusetts. The law requires statewide industries to disclose the chemicals they use, and since its passage the state's environmental emissions decreased by 73 percent. This could set the stage for phasing out harmful carcinogens.

The effort to reform NCI will closely monitor how it spends its annual budget of some $4.6 billion. Tracking NCI's budget increases against the cancer incidence numbers. The more money we spend on cancer, the more cancer we get.

NCI should be doing more research on avoidable exposures to industrial carcinogens and should inform the public of known risks from occupational and environmental exposure to carcinogens.

This research could complement the available data on air and water pollutants documented through the U.S. Environmental Protection Agency's National Toxic Release Inventory as well as data from states.

"We have not begun to win the war on cancer," said Dr. Richard Clapp, an epidemiological professor at the Boston University School of Public Health. "We have not even turned the corner. We have to move beyond the body count and begin to prevent exposures before they occur."

ENDORSERS:

Dr. Richard Clapp
Boston University

Dr. Nicholas Ashford
Massachusetts Institute of Technology

NATIONAL CANCER INSTITUTE LEADERSHIP IS OUT OF TOUCH WITH REALITY

In a February 11, 2003 speech to an advisory board, Andrew von Eschenbach, the Director of the National Cancer Institute (NCI), pledged to eliminate "the suffering and death" from cancer by 2015. He stated: "I have set out . . . a challenge goal that shapes our mission and shapes our vision . . . to eliminate the suffering and death due to cancer, and to do it by 2015."

Dr. von Eschenbach's goal is irresponsible and unrealistic warned Samuel S. Epstein, M.D. What is the possible scientific basis for such claims? "Does Dr. von Eschenbach know something no one else knows? Is he familiar with the NCI data on incidence and mortality? What great advances or breakthroughs does he know, of which no one else is aware? Has he been talking with God?

Since 1971, the overall incidence of cancer has escalated to epidemic proportions, now striking about 1.3 million and killing about 550,000 annually; nearly one in two men and more than one in three women now develop cancer in their lifetimes. While smoking is unquestionably the single largest cause of cancer, the incidence of lung cancer in men has declined sharply. In striking contrast, there have been major increases in the incidence of a wide range of non-smoking cancers in men and women, and also of childhood cancers.

The current cancer epidemic does not reflect lack of resources. Paradoxically, NCI's escalating budget is paralleled by the escalating incidence of cancer. Since 1971, NCI's budget has increased approximately 30-fold, from $220 million to $4.6 billion.

According to the Cancer Prevention Coalition, the fundamental reason why we are losing the winnable war against cancer is because NCI's mindset is fixated on damage control-screening, diagnosis, and treatment-and basic research. This is coupled with indifference to preventing a wide range of avoidable exposures to industrial carcinogens, contaminating the totality of the environment—air, water, and soil—the workplace, and consumer products—food, cosmetics and toiletries and household products. This denial of the public's right-to-know of such avoidable cancer risks is in contrast to NCI's stream of press releases, briefings, and media reports claiming the latest advances in treatment and basic research.

The silence of the NCI on avoidable causes of cancer has tacitly encouraged corporate polluters and industries to continue manufacturing and marketing carcinogenic products. This silence also violates amendments of the National Cancer Act, calling for "an expanded and intensified research program for the prevention of cancer caused by occupational or environmental exposure to carcinogens."

Nevertheless, NCI's prevention policies are virtually restricted to faulty lifestyle considerations. As strikingly exemplified in von Eschenbach's recent speech, prevention is defined only in terms of tobacco, "energy balance" and obesity. However, this is hardly surprising as von Eschenbach was President-Elect of the ACS prior to his appointment as NCI Director. The ACS Cancer Facts and Figures 2002 dismissively reassures that carcinogenic exposures from dietary pesticides, "toxic wastes in dump sites," ionizing radiation from "closely controlled" nuclear power plants, and non-ionizing radiation, are all "at such low levels that risks are negligible."

Dr. von Eschenbach also remained Director of the ACS 1998 National Dialogue on Cancer, which seeks a major role in federal cancer policies. It may be further noted that The Chronicle of Philanthropy, the nation's leading charity watch dog, has charged that the ACS "is more interested in accumulating wealth than saving lives."

These concerns are detailed in the Cancer Prevention Coalition (CPC) report, "Stop Cancer Before It Starts Campaign: How to Win the Losing War Against Cancer," released at a Feb. 20 Washington, D.C., press conference. This report is endorsed by some 100 leading cancer prevention scientists, public health and policy experts, and representatives of concerned citizen groups, who advocate major reforms of national cancer policies.

March 27, 2003

ENVIRONMENTAL CAUSES OF CANCER NEGLECTED

Despite hugely increased funding for cancer research and prevention, the overall incidence of cancer in the United States has escalated to epidemic proportions in the last three decades. It now strikes about 1.3 million people and kills about 550,000 each year: nearly one in two men and more than one in three women now develop cancer in their lifetimes. The problem is that environmental causes have been largely ignored.

While smoking is unquestionably the single largest cause of lung cancer, besides a risk factor for some other cancers, the incidence of lung and other smoking-related cancers in US men has declined sharply. In striking contrast, there has been a major increase in the incidence of predominantly non-smoking cancers in men and women, especially among blacks, and also in childhood cancers. This increase in cancer and especially in non-smoking cancers, is reflected in the United Kingdom and other major industrialized nations.

Nevertheless, the US National Cancer Institute (NCI) has repeatedly made misleading assurances of major progress in the war against cancer for over two decades. NCI's 1998 Report Card, claimed a recent "reversal of an almost 20-year trend of increasing cancer cases." However, this "reversal" was minimal and misleading. In October 2002, NCI admitted to significant errors in underestimating its published incidence data, apart from delays in reporting these data. Against this background, NCI Director Andrew von Eschenbach's February 2003 pledge to "eliminate the suffering and death due to cancer . . . and to do it by 2015" seem incongruous.

The escalating incidence of cancer does not reflect lack of resources. Since 1970, NCI's budget has increased approximately 30-fold, reaching $4.6 billion for 2003. Paradoxically, NCI's escalating budget over the last three decades is paralleled by the escalating incidence of cancer.

Apart from basic research, NCI's mindset remains fixated on "secondary" prevention or damage control—screening, diagnosis, and chemoprevention (the use of drugs or nutrients to reduce risks from prior avoidable carcinogenic exposures)—and treatment. This is coupled with indifference to primary prevention, preventing a wide range of avoidable, environmental causes of cancer, other than faulty lifestyle: smoking, inactivity, and fatty diet.

The decades-long silence of NCI on a wide range of avoidable causes of cancer, other than personal lifestyle, has tacitly encouraged powerful corporate polluters and industries manufacturing carcinogenic products. Such corporate conduct has been characterized, "white collar crime," by Congressman J. Conyers in his 1979 and 1984 Bills, intended to extend such legislation to economically motivated crimes with adverse public health or environmental consequences. The NCI is thus complicit in these adverse public health consequences, and bears heavy responsibility for losing the winnable war against cancer and for the current cancer epidemic.

National cancer policies are now threatened more than ever before by NCI's indifference to primary prevention, and its silence on avoidable causes of cancer, other than personal lifestyle. As seriously, this silence reflects denial of citizens' democratic Right-to-Know and empowerment, and rejection of environmental justice, by sacrificing citizens' health and welfare to powerful corporate interests.

The war against cancer must be fought by strategies based on primary prevention, rather than reactively on secondary prevention or damage control. As importantly, this war must be waged by leadership accountable to the public and not special interests.

ENDORSER:

Quentin D. Young, MD
Chairman of Health and Medicine Policy Research Group
Past President of the American Public Health Association

November 4, 2003

AN OUNCE OF PREVENTION

Cancer has become the leading cause of disease and death in the United States. A much higher priority for prevention would reduce this carnage, and the need for treatment.

In 1971, Congress passed the National Cancer Act and Program. This was prompted by well orchestrated appeals from leading representatives of the "cancer establishment," the federal National Cancer Institute (NCI) and the world's wealthiest nonprofit organization, the American Cancer Society (ACS). They promised that the cure for cancer was imminent, but only if given an increase in NCI's funding.

Spurred on by a major media campaign, aggressively promoted by NCI and ACS representatives, including a full page advertisement in "The New York Times," "Mr. Nixon, You Can Cure Cancer," President Richard Nixon enthusiastically embraced the Act. He launched the "War Against Cancer," increased NCI's 1971 budget from $150 to $220 million, and gave NCI unprecedented autonomy.

Unfortunately, the Act had unintended consequences. The Act authorized the President to appoint the director of the NCI, and authorize its budget, thus bypassing the director of all the other 26 National Institutes of Health. The Act thus effectively insulated and politicized the National Cancer Institute.

Over 30 years and some $55 billion later, we are further away from winning the cancer war than when it was first declared. But that is contrary to what we had been led to believe.

Since passage of the 1971 Act, the National Cancer Institute and the ACS have reassured the nation with a steady stream of misleading press releases, briefings, and media reports hailing major progress in the cancer war.

These include repeated claims for miracle "breakthroughs" in cancer treatment, and also the 1984 and 1986 NCI promises that cancer mortality would be halved by 2000.

The misleading statements include the 1998 reassurances by the NCI and ACS that the nation had "turned the corner" in the war on cancer, and the February 11, 2003 incredible "pledge" by NCI director Dr. Andrew von Eschenbach to "eliminate the suffering and death from cancer by 2015."

Also misleading is the September 2003 claim, in the "Annual Report to the Nation on the Status of Cancer, 1975-2000," by the NCI, co-authored by the

ACS, and the Centers for Disease Control and Prevention, that "considerable progress has been made in reducing the burden of cancer."

These claims don't even pass the laugh test. Cancer mortality rates have remained virtually unchanged (199/100,000) from 1975 to 2000. These rates are based on NCI's statistics, which are adjusted to compensate for the aging population.

Over the same period, overall cancer incidence rates have escalated by 18 percent, now striking about 1.3 million annually. Today, nearly one in two men and more than one in three women develop cancer in their lifetimes.

This translates into approximately 56 percent more cancer in men, and 22 percent more cancer in women over the course of a single generation. Cancer has become a disease of "mass destruction."

Contrary to what one might think, this increase is not due to smoking. Lung cancer rates have dropped sharply due to decreased smoking by men over recent decades.

Furthermore, the increased incidence rates from 1975 to 2000 involve many cancers unrelated to smoking. These include: non-Hodgkin's lymphoma (71 percent); testes (54 percent); thyroid (54 percent); breast (29 percent); and acute myeloid leukemia (15 percent). For African Americans, cancer rates are even higher, with excesses up to 120 percent.

Childhood cancers now strike about 9,000 young people each year and are killing about 1,500 annually. From 1975 to 2000, childhood cancer rates have increased dramatically. These include: acute lymphocytic leukemia (59 percent), brain cancer (48 percent), kidney cancer (43 percent), and bone cancer (20 percent).

The escalating incidence of childhood and non-smoking related adult cancers is paralleled by NCI's escalating budget from $220 million in 1971 to the current $4.6 billion, a 30-fold increase.

Paradoxically, it seems that the more we spend on cancer, the more cancer we get.

The reason why we are losing the winnable cancer war is because the cancer establishment's priorities remain fixated on damage control—screening, diagnosis, and treatment—and related basic research.

All these are unarguably important, and deserve substantial funding. However, much less funding would be needed if more cancer was prevented, with less cancer to treat.

The pro-industry agenda of the American Cancer Society is exemplified by its minuscule prevention research budget. In spite of bloated contrary claims, less than 0.1 percent of its $800 million budget has been allocated to research on the prevention of environmental carcinogenesis.

ACS' financial ties to the cancer drug and polluting industries remain extensive. Over 25 drug and biotech companies are Excalibur donors, who each have contributed in excess of $100,000 annually. These include: Bristol-Myers Squibb, Pfizer, AstraZeneca, Eli Lilly, Amgen, Genentech, and Johnson & Johnson.

Polluting industries that are donors include over 10 petrochemical and oil companies, such as British Petroleum, DuPont, Akzo Nobel, Pennzoil and Concho Oil. Other donors include global cosmetic companies, such as Elizabeth Arden, Revlon, Christian Dior, and Givaudan.

A total of some 300 other industries and companies make similar contributions to ACS's $800 million annual budget, a figure that excludes government grants, and income from about $1 billion in reserves. These figures hardly justify annual appeals, claiming the need for more funds to continue support of ongoing cancer programs.

As might be anticipated, the ACS returns its donors' favors with more than a wink and a nod. The society has supported the automobile industry in refusing to endorse the Clean Air Act. It has joined the Chlorine Institute in defending the continued manufacture of chlorinated carcinogenic pesticides. And it has supported the cosmetic industry in failing to warn women of risks of breast and other cancers from permanent black hair dyes, and of risks of ovarian cancer from sanitary dusting with talc.

Not surprisingly, "The Chronicle of Philanthropy," the nation's leading charity watchdog, charged in 1992 that, "The ACS is more interested in accumulating wealth than saving lives." The Chronicle also warned against the transfer of money from the public purse to private hands.

The most disturbing development in the cancer war has been its privatization by the ACS. In 1998, the ACS created and funded the National Dialogue on Cancer (NDC), co-chaired by former President George Bush, and Barbara Bush. Included were a wide range of cancer survivor groups, some 100 representatives of the cancer drug industry, and Shandwick International PR, whose major clients include R.J. Reynolds Tobacco Holdings.

In the *Cancer Letter*, an insider cancer publication which has investigated the NDC from its onset, Dr. Durant charged the ACS with "protecting their own fund raising capacity . . . from competition by survivor groups. It has always seemed to me that this was an issue of control by the ACS over the cancer agenda."

Without informing NDC's participants, and behind closed doors, the American Cancer Society then spun off a small Legislative Committee. Its explicit objective was to advise Congress on the need to replace the 1971 National Cancer Act with a new National Cancer Control Act. The new Act is intended to shift major control of cancer policy from the public National Cancer Institute to the nonprofit American Cancer Society.

The proposed Act would also increase NCI funding from this year's $4.6 billion to $14 billion by 2007. The American Cancer Society was assisted by Shandwick in drafting the new Act and managing the National Dialogue on Cancer.

Following the embarrassing January 2000 disclosure that R.J. Reynolds Tobacco Holdings was one of Shandwick's major clients, about which the ACS claimed it has been unaware, the PR firm was promptly fired.

But then, ACS hired another well known tobacco PR firm, Edelman Public Relations Worldwide, to conduct a voter cancer education campaign for the 2000 Presidential elections.

Edelman represents the Brown & Williamson Tobacco Company, and The Altria Group, the parent company of Philip Morris, the nation's biggest cigarette maker.

With the February 2002 appointment of ACS President-Elect von Eschenbach as National Cancer Institute director, the National Cancer Program was effectively privatized.

Commenting on the ACS relationship with the tobacco industry, prominent anti-smoking activist Dr. Stanton Glantz said, "It's like . . . Bush hiring Al Qaeda to do PR, because they have good connections to Al-Jazeera."

Playing the other side of the coin, on August 19 the ACS announced strong support for increasing the Food and Drug Administration's authority to regulate tobacco products.

Meanwhile, the good cop/bad cop relationship between the ACS and the tobacco industry and other polluting industries continues to escape public attention.

As disturbing is the growing secretive collaboration between the NCI and the ACS-NDC complex, as revealed in the August 2003 Cancer Letter.

The latest example is the joint planning of a massive tumor tissue bank. This would cost between $500 million and $1.2 billion to operate, apart from construction costs in the billions.

This initiative would be privatized, rife with conflicts of interest, exempt from the provisions of the Federal Advisory Committee and Freedom of Information Acts, and free from federal technology transfer regulations.

These developments, coupled with the NCI's track record on prevention, fully justify the recommendations of the July 2003 report by The National Academy of Sciences (NAS).

The report stressed the autonomous "special status" of the NCI, resulting in "an unnecessary rift between (its) goals and leadership" and those of the National Institutes of Health.

More seriously, control of the nation's cancer agenda has been surreptitiously transferred from the public to the private sector's special interests.

A Congressional investigation of these critical concerns, and NCI's failure to implement the National Cancer Act's mandate is decades overdue.

ENDORSER:

Quentin D. Young, MD
Chairman of the Health and Medicine Policy Research Group
Past President of the American Public Health Association.

February 23, 2004

SPINNING THE LOSING CANCER WAR

In politics, spinning is an art form. Most accept spinning as a fact of life, whether choosing a politician or merely a bar of soap. However, few would accept this gamesmanship for life and death issues of cancer, particularly if the spinning is underwritten by taxpayers.

But, when it comes to the cancer war, the Pollyannaish promises of the federal National Cancer Institute (NCI) and the non-profit American Cancer Society (ACS) are no more reliable than political flack.

Recent headlines in national newspapers, based on NCI and ACS assurances, report that the "Rate of Cancer Deaths Continues to Drop." This reinforces long-standing claims of miracle "breakthrough" treatments, that mortality would be halved by 2000, that the nation had "turned the corner" in the cancer war, and that "considerable progress has been made in reducing the burden of cancer." However, these claims don't even pass the laugh test.

Cancer death rates have remained unchanged since President Nixon declared the 1971 War Against Cancer. Nearly one in two men, and more than one in three women are now struck by cancer. Cancer has become a disease of "mass destruction."

Contrary to the NCI and ACS, the current cancer epidemic is not due to faulty lifestyle—smoking, unhealthy diet, and obesity. American men smoke less today, and lung cancer rates are steadily dropping. In striking contrast, the incidence of environmentally, and non-smoking related cancers has escalated sharply: non-Hodgkin's lymphoma by 71 percent, testes and thyroid cancers by 54 percent each, post-menopausal breast cancer by 37 percent, and myeloid leukemia by 15 percent; various childhood cancers have increased from 20 to 60 percent. For African Americans, the news is worse: incidence rates have increased by up to 120 percent

The escalating incidence of non-smoking adult cancers and childhood cancers is paralleled by the 30-fold increase in NCI's budget from $220 million in 1972 to the current $4.6 billion. The ACS budget has increased from $130 to $800 million, with about $1 billion in reserves. It seems that the more we spend on cancer, the more cancer we get.

The reason we are losing this winnable war is because NCI and ACS priorities remain fixated on damage control—screening, diagnosis, and treatment—and related basic research. All merit substantial funding.

However, less funding would be needed if more cancer was prevented, with less to treat.

Responding to criticisms of such imbalanced priorities, NCI now allocates 12 percent of its budget to "prevention and control," and requires its nationwide Centers to have a "prevention component." However, cancer prevention continues to be narrowly defined in terms of faulty lifestyle, and screening, and excludes any reference to avoidable causes of cancer from exposures to industrial carcinogens. These include: contaminants of air, water, food, and the workplace; ingredients in cosmetics and toiletries, and household products, particularly pesticides.

NCI's indifference to such avoidable causes of cancer extends to denial. For example, NCI claims that, "The causes of childhood cancer are largely unknown," in spite of substantial contrary evidence. Similarly, ACS reassures that carcinogenic exposures from dietary pesticides, "toxic wastes in dump sites," and radiation from "closely controlled" nuclear power plants are all "at such low levels that risks are negligible."

Not surprisingly, Congressman John Conyers (D-MI), Ranking Member of the House Judiciary Committee and Dean of the Congressional Black Caucus, recently warned that so much cancer carnage is preventable. "Preventable, that is if the NCI gets off the dime and does its job."

NCI and ACS policies are compounded by conflicts of interest, particularly with the cancer drug industry. In a 1998 Washington Post interview, Dr. Samuel Broder, NCI's former Director, dropped a bombshell: "The NCI has become what amounts to a government pharmaceutical company." Broder resigned from the NCI to become successive Chief Officer of two major cancer drugs companies.

The ACS has a fund raising apparatus which would make any Presidential candidate blush. Apart from public donations, the ACS swims in the largesse of over 300 Excalibur industry donors, each contributing over $100,000 annually. These include over 25 drug and biotech companies, and petrochemical and oil industries. Unbelievably, ACS legislative initiatives are handled by Edelman PR, the major lobbyist of the tobacco industry, and fast food and beverage companies, now targeted by anti-obesity litigation.

Not surprisingly, The Chronicle of Philanthropy, the nation's leading charity watchdog, has charged: "The ACS is more interested in accumulating wealth than saving lives."

The cancer war is certainly winnable, given radical changes in its high command and priorities, and given information on avoidable industrial causes of cancer is provided to the public and Congress. The President has finally conceded the need for an independent commission to investigate misrepresentations that led us into the war on Iraq. We should use a similar commission to investigate the much more lethal failure of the cancer war.

ENDORSER:

Quentin D. Young, MD
Chairman of the Health & Medicine Policy Research Group
Past President of the American Public Health Association

April 27, 2005

CANCER WAR SHOULD FOCUS ON PREVENTION

Today, there are generals waging a war that continues to take a massive toll of Americans' health and life. These generals are asking for billions of dollars—on top of the more than $50 billion already spent—to defeat the enemy's scourge. But increasingly, independent experts are reporting that the generals' intelligence and strategies are patently wrong, and that they consciously misrepresent critical facts in order to paint false, rosy scenarios.

In all likelihood, you must suspect that I am referring to the Iraq war. But there is actually another war being handled with startling ham-handedness and deception. It's a war that claims far more victims than the war against terror. It is the war against cancer.

In 1971, President Nixon declared the war against cancer and Congress passed the National Cancer Act. These actions ushered in the new battle, spurring a 30-fold increase in the budget of the government's National Cancer Institute—to a tune of $5 billion this year. The new war also helped the nation's leading cancer charity, the American Cancer Society, raise tens of millions in public donations.

With the wind at their backs, and locked at the hip, leaders of the NCI and ACS became the generals in the new war, and have spent billions of tax and public dollars in waging it over ensuing years.

But after three decades of highly publicized and misleading promises of progress, the sad reality has finally dawned: We are in fact losing the cancer war, in what can only be described as a rout. The incidence of cancers—notably breast, testes, thyroid, myeloma, lymphomas and childhood—all unrelated to smoking—has escalated to epidemic proportions, now striking nearly one in every two men, and more than one in every three women. Meanwhile, overall mortality rates—the indicator of our ability to survive cancer once it strikes—have remained unchanged for decades.

There is strong scientific evidence that this epidemic is due to avoidable exposures to industrial carcinogens in the totality of the environment—air, water, soil, workplaces as well as consumer products, notably, food, toiletries and cosmetics and household products—and even some common prescription drugs.

But our ongoing defeat in this war is attributable to two important factors.

First, NCI and ACS have focused their abundant resources and institutional mind-sets not on preventing cancer, but on attempting to treat it once it strikes. NCI, for instance, allocates less than an estimated 3 percent of its budget to environmental causes of cancer, while the ACS allocates less than 0.1 percent toward this goal. As recently admitted by the president of one of NCI's leading cancer centers, most NCI resources are spent on "promoting ineffective drugs" for terminal disease.

By forsaking prevention—the basic principle that medicine has taught us over the centuries, and the need for which science again underscores in the war against cancer—our cancer generals have embraced a "damage-control" strategy, akin to treating wounded soldiers, rather than trying to halt further advance of the enemy.

The simple fact—the more cancer is prevented, the less there is to treat—continues to elude the generals' master plan.

Another reason why our cancer generals are so disserving is that they have become far too chummy with special interests who either oppose cancer prevention policies or who trivialize cancer prevention. The ACS heavily depends on their "Excalibur donors"—a gallery of chemical industries opposed to regulating carcinogens, and pharmaceutical companies seeking approval of their highly touted miracle drugs—drugs that have shown limited if any success over decades.

Similarly the NCI has also developed incestuous relationships with cancer drug companies. Indeed, a former NCI director candidly admitted that the NCI "has become what amounts to a governmental pharmaceutical company."

In order to change course, drastic reforms are needed in the cancer war high command and strategies. Both NCI and ACS must be required to devote at least equal priority and resources to prevent as to treat cancer. The NCI and ACS must also be required to inform the public, Congress and regulatory agencies of substantial scientific evidence on industrial, and other avoidable causes of cancer. Congress should also ensure that companies that pollute our environment and consumer products with industrial carcinogens are held to the highest standards of accountability and disclosure.

Nearly every American knows the pain to family and friends caused by cancer. The crime is that so much of it is avoidable.

April 2, 2007

THE UNITED NATIONS TAKES THE INITIATIVE IN THE WAR AGAINST CANCER

This week, after notables such as Elizabeth Edwards and Tony Snow, have shared the bad news with the nation that their cancers have returned, we are deluged with a series of editorials in last Sunday's New York Times. These emphasize early screening, the latest promise of new treatment modalities, and the latest promise of new genetic research. However, not once in any of these editorials or other news items is the word prevention even mentioned.

Rather than winning the cancer war, we have been losing it progressively since President Richard Nixon declared the War on Cancer in 1971. Today, cancer strikes nearly 1.3 million people annually. Nearly one in two men and more than one in three women develop cancer in their lifetimes. This translates into approximately 56 percent more cancer in men and 22 percent more cancer in women over the course of just one generation.

Since 1971, and with some $50 billion taxpayers funding of the National Cancer Institute, the incidence of a wide range of cancers unrelated to smoking has escalated to near epidemic proportions. These include: thyroid cancer by over 80%; childhood leukemia by 70%; non-Hodgkin's lymphoma by 70%; and testes cancer by 50%.

More disturbingly, there is long-standing, well-documented epidemiological evidence on the avoidable causes of these cancers, notably environmental and occupational carcinogens. There is also well documented evidence on carcinogenic ingredients and contaminants in common consumer products-food, cosmetics and personal care products, and household products.

However, this evidence is ignored or trivialized by the National Cancer Institute in lock step with the world's largest charity, the American Cancer Society. This charity has been characterized by The Chronicle of Philanthropy, the nation's leading charity watchdog, as "more interested in accumulating wealth than saving lives."

Responding to these critical concerns, the United Nations has just announced a critical initiative on "Meeting the Global Challenge of Cancer." This has been created in response to the World Health Organization's warning that "We are now on the brink of an international cancer epidemic, with cancer now representing far more deaths than HIV, AIDS, tuberculosis, and malaria combined."

The United Nations has recently invited Dr. Samuel S. Epstein and Dr. Nicholas Ashford to take a lead role in launching its Stop Cancer initiative, and on how to win the losing cancer war, an invitation we have readily accepted.

ENDORSER:

Nicholas A. Ashford, PhD, JD
Professor of Technology and Policy
Director, MIT Technology and Law Program
Massachusetts Institute of Technology

December 2, 2008

THE OBAMA CANCER PLAN

Obama is the first President-elect to develop a comprehensive cancer plan, besides doubling cancer funding. While the plan reflects strong emphasis on oncology, no reference is made to cancer prevention.

The plan defines and coordinates the responsibilities of four federal agencies: the National Cancer Institute (NCI), for research and clinical trials; the Centers for Disease Control and Prevention, for epidemiological follow up and support of cancer survivors; the Centers for Medicare and Medicaid Services, for funding cancer related care; and the FDA, for regulating cancer drugs.

In 1971, Congress passed the National Cancer Act which authorized the National Cancer Program, calling for "an expanded and intensified research program for the prevention of cancer caused by occupational or environmental exposures to carcinogens." Shortly afterwards, President Nixon announced his "War Against Cancer," and authorized a $200 million budget for the NCI. Since then, its budget has escalated by nearly 30-fold, to $5.3 billion this year.

Meanwhile, the incidence of a wide range of cancers, other than those due to smoking, has escalated sharply from 1971 to 2005, when the latest NCI statistics were published. These include malignant melanoma (170%), Non-Hodgkin's lymphoma (80%), thyroid (117%), testis (60%), and childhood cancers (10%).

As widely reported in the November 26, 2008, press, the NCI, and the American Cancer Society now claim that the incidence of new cancers has been falling from 1999 to 2005. However, this is contrary to NCI's latest statistics. These show increases of 45% for thyroid cancer, 18% for malignant melanoma, 18% for kidney cancer, 10% for childhood cancers, and 4% for testes cancer.

Disturbingly, the NCI has still failed to develop, let alone publicize, any listing or registry of avoidable exposures to a wide range of carcinogens. These include: some pharmaceuticals; diagnostic radiation; occupational; environmental; and ingredients in consumer products-food, household products, and cosmetics and personal care products. The NCI has also failed to respond, other than misleadingly or dismissively, to prior Congressional requests for such information.

In March 1998, in a series of questions to then NCI Director Dr. Richard Klausner, Cong. David Obey requested information on NCI's policies and priorities. These included whether "Other than tobacco and sunlight, . . . the general public has been adequately informed about avoidable causes of cancer?"

The answer was, and remains, no. Klausner's response made it clear that NCI persisted in indifference to cancer prevention, coupled with imbalanced emphasis on damage control-diagnosis, treatment, and clinical trials.

Moreover, NCI's claims for the success of "innovative treatment" have been sharply criticized by distinguished oncologists. In 2004, Nobelist Leland Hartwell, President of the Fred Hutchinson Cancer Control Center, warned that "Congress and the public are not paying NCI $5 billion a year, most of which is spent on promoting ineffective drugs for terminal disease."

It should be further emphasized that the costs of new biotech cancer drugs have increased approximately 500-fold over the last decade. Furthermore, the U.S. spends five times more than the U.K. on chemotherapy per patient, although their survival rates are similar.

The re-election of Congressman Obey to head the House Appropriations Subcommittee is welcome news. In this role, he is in a position to strengthen Obama's cancer plan by emphasizing that the more cancer is prevented, the less there is to treat.

January 23, 2009

OBAMA CANCER PLAN MUST PRIORITIZE PREVENTION

President Barack Obama is the first President to develop a comprehensive cancer plan. While the plan reflects strong emphasis on oncology, the diagnosis and treatment of cancer, no reference is made to prevention. Yet, the more cancer that can be prevented, the less there is to treat.

President Obama's cancer plan should emphasize the many avoidable causes of cancer.

The plan defines and coordinates the responsibilities of four federal agencies: the National Cancer Institute (NCI), for research and clinical trials; the Centers for Disease Control and Prevention, for epidemiological follow up and support of cancer survivors; the Centers for Medicare & Medicaid Services, for funding cancer related care; and the FDA, for regulating cancer drugs.

In 1971, Congress passed the National Cancer Act which authorized the National Cancer Program, calling for an expanded and intensified research program for the prevention of cancer caused by occupational or environmental exposures to carcinogens. Shortly afterwards, President Richard Nixon announced his "War Against Cancer," and authorized a $200 million budget for the NCI. Since then, its budget has escalated by nearly 30-fold, to $5.3 billion this year.

Meanwhile, the incidence of a wide range of cancers, other than those due to smoking, has escalated sharply from 1975 to 2005, when the latest NCI statistics were published. These include malignant melanoma (172%), Non-Hodgkin's lymphoma (79%), thyroid (116%), testes (60%), and childhood cancers (38%).

In November 2008, the NCI claimed that the incidence of new cancers has been falling from 1999 to 2005. However, this is contrary to its own latest statistics. These show increases of 45% for thyroid cancer, 18% for malignant melanoma, 18% for kidney cancer, 10% for childhood cancers, and 4% for testes cancer.

Disturbingly, the NCI has still failed to develop, let alone publicize, any listing or registry of avoidable exposures to a wide range of carcinogens. These include: some pharmaceuticals; high dose diagnostic radiation; occupational; environmental; and ingredients in consumer products—food, household products, and cosmetics and personal care products.

The NCI has also failed to respond, other than misleadingly or dismissively, to prior Congressional requests for such information.

In March 1998, in a series of questions to then NCI Director Dr. Richard Klausner, Congressman David Obey requested information on NCI's policies and priorities. He asked, "Should the NCI develop a registry of avoidable carcinogens and make this information widely available to the public?" The answer was, and remains, no.

Klausner's responses made it clear that NCI persisted in indifference to cancer prevention, coupled with imbalanced emphasis on damage control—screening, diagnosis, treatment, and clinical trials.

Moreover, NCI's claims for the success of "innovative treatment" have been sharply criticized by distinguished oncologists. In 2004, Nobelist Leland Hartwell, President of the Fred Hutchinson Cancer Control Center, warned that "Congress and the public are not paying NCI $4.7 billion a year, most of which is spent on promoting ineffective drugs" for terminal disease.

It should be further emphasized that the costs of new biotech cancer drugs have increased more than 100-fold over the last decade. Furthermore, the U.S. spends five times more than the U.K. on chemotherapy per patient, although their survival rates are similar.

The Obama Cancer Plan is subject to Congressional authorization, and funding approval by the House and Senate Appropriations Committees. These committees will be in a position to require that major priority should be directed to cancer prevention rather than to oncology. Clearly, the more cancer is prevented, the less there is to treat. This will also be of major help in achieving Obama's goal "to lower health care costs."

This release has been endorsed by ninteen leading national experts in cancer prevention. They are as follows:

Nicholas A. Ashford, PhD, JD
Professor of Technology and Policy
Director, MIT Technology and Law Program
Massachusetts Institute of Technology
Cambridge, Massachusetts

Rosalie Bertell, PhD
International Association for Humanitarian Medicine
International Science Oversight Committee for the Organic Consumers Association
Yardley, Pennsylvania

James Brophy, PhD
Adjunct Assistant Professor
Department of Sociology and Anthropology
Board of Directors, Toxic Free Canada
University of Windsor
Ontario, Canada

Richard Clapp, DSc, MPH
Professor
Boston University School of Public Health
Boston, Massachusetts

Paul Connett, PhD
Professor Emeritus of Environmental Chemistry,
St. Lawrence University
Canton, New York;
Executive Director
Fluoride Action Network
Canton, New York

Ronnie Cummins
National Director
Organic Consumers Association
Finland, Minnesota

Tracey Easthope, MPH
Director, Environmental Health Project
Ecology Center
Ann Arbor, Michigan

Lennart Hardell, MD, PhD
Professor
Department of Oncology
University Hospital
Orebro, Sweden

Hazel Henderson, DSc Hon., FRSA, author, futurist
President, Ethical Markets Media, LLC;
Co-Creator, the Calvert Group of the Calvert-Henderson Quality of
Life Indicators

Margaret Keith, PhD
Adjunct Assistant Professor
Department of Sociology and Anthropology
Board of Directors Toxic Free Canada
University of Windsor
Ontario, Canada

Joseph Mangano, MPH, MBA
Executive Director
Radiation and Public Health Project
New York, New York

James R. Mellow, MD, MS
Robert Wood Johnson Family Medicine Fellow
Physicians for Social Responsibility
Alliance for a Clean and Healthy Maine
Portland, Maine

Vicente Navarro, MD, PhD
Professor of Health Policy
The Johns Hopkins Medical Institutions
Baltimore, Maryland

Peter Orris, MD, MPH, FACP, FACOEM
Professor and Chief of Service
Environmental and Occupational Medicine
University of Illinois at Chicago Medical Center;
Professor, Internal and Preventive Medicine
Rush University College of Medicine;
Professor, Preventive Medicine
Northwestern University Feinberg School of Medicine
Chicago, Illinois

Lawrence A. Plumlee, MD
President, Chemical Sensitivity Disorders Association
Bethesda, Maryland

Horst Rechelbacher
President, Intelligent Nutrients
Minneapolis, Minnesota

Janette D. Sherman, MD
Adjunct Professor Environmental Institute
Western Michigan University
Kalamazoo, Michigan

Eileen M. Wright, MD, ABIHM
Great Smokies Medical Center
Asheville, North Carolina

Daphne Wysham
Fellow, Institute for Policy Studies
Washington, District of Columbia

Quentin D. Young, MD
Chairman, Health and Medicine Policy Research Group
Chicago, Illinois

June 15, 2009

MEDICAL EXPERTS PRESCRIBE LEGISLATION TO HELP PREVENT CANCER

A letter to Congressional leaders urging drastic revision of the Obama Cancer Plan to mandate prevention was released today by medical and scientific experts on the causes and prevention of cancer.

The letter expressing their concern that cancer prevention has received no attention in the Obama plan is addressed to four congressional committees: the Senate Committee on Health, Education, Labor and Pensions; the Senate Appropriations Committee; the House Committee on Energy and Commerce; and the House Appropriations Committee.

The experts recommend that Congress enact legislative reforms to the 1971 National Cancer Act, including a statement that it is the national policy of the United States to reduce carcinogenic exposures by at least half during the next decade. They also urge the annual publication of a comprehensive public register of carcinogens.

The scientists and doctors prescribe major policy changes for the National Cancer Institute (NCI). These include the appointment of a new Deputy Director for Cancer Prevention, and the allocation of at least 40% of the NCI budget to prevention programs for Fiscal Year 2011.

The text of the letter follows.

> Senator Edward M. Kennedy
> Chairman, Senate Committee on Health, Education, Labor and Pensions
>
> Senator Mike Enzi
> Ranking Member, Senate Committee on Health, Education, Labor and Pensions
>
> Senator Daniel K. Inouye
> Chairman, Senate Committee on Appropriations
>
> Senator Thad Cochran
> Ranking Member, Senate Committee on Appropriations
>
> Representative Henry A. Waxman
> Chairman, House Committee on Energy and Commerce

Representative Joe Barton
Ranking Member, House Committee on Energy and Commerce

Representative David Obey
Chairman, House Committee on Appropriations

Representative Jerry Lewis
Ranking Member, House Committee on Appropriations

Dear Senators and Representatives;

President Obama has boldly pledged to reform the national health care system. Central to this, as the president has stressed, is containing the spiraling costs of health care—costs which are soaring at about 6% each year. Most experts agree that this is not possible without a better plan to prevent Americans from getting cancer in the first place. This year, 1.5 million people will be diagnosed with cancer. Of them, 562,000 people—over 1,500 every day—will die.

The cancer epidemic strikes as many as one in three Americans and takes the life of one in four. After 37 years of losing the war against cancer (a war that President Nixon originally declared in December 1971), we are taking grossly and demonstrably inadequate action to protect us from this menace.

While research on the prevention and treatment of cancer is predominantly the responsibility of the National Cancer Institute (NCI), other governmental agencies are also involved. These include the Environmental Protection Agency (EPA), the Occupational Safety and Health Administration (OSHA), the Consumer Product Safety Commission (CPSC), and the Food and Drug Administration (FDA). Unfortunately, such action is uncoordinated and unbalanced.

The connection between our losing the cancer war and the need to control costs through prevention is clear. Cancer is not only one of the most costly and sometimes deadly diseases in America, it is also one of the most preventable.

Based on recent estimates by the National Institutes of Health, the total costs of cancer are $219 billion a year. The annual costs to taxpayers of diagnosis and treatment amount to $89 billion; the annual costs of premature death are conservatively estimated at $112 billion; and the annual costs due to lost productivity are conservatively estimated at $18 billion. And these are the quantifiable, inflationary economic costs. The human costs surely are of far greater magnitude.

To be sure, smoking remains the best-known and single largest cause of cancer, particularly lung cancer. While incidence rates of lung cancer in men have declined by 20% over the past three decades, rates in women increased by

111%. But more importantly, non-smoking cancers—due to known chemical and physical carcinogens—have increased substantially since 1975. Some of the more startling realities in the failure to prevent cancer are illustrated by their soaring rates of increase. These include:

- Malignant melanoma of the skin in adults is increasing by 168% due to the use of sunscreens in childhood that fail to block long wave ultraviolet light;
- Thyroid cancer is increasing by 124% due in large part to ionizing radiation;
- Non-Hodgkin's lymphoma is increasing 76% due mostly to phenoxy herbicides; and phenylenediamine hair dyes;
- Testicular cancer is increasing by 49% due to pesticides; hormonal ingredients in cosmetics and personal care products; and estrogen residues in meat;
- Childhood leukemia is increasing by 55% due to ionizing radiation; domestic pesticides; nitrite preservatives in meats, particularly hot dogs; and parental exposures to occupational carcinogens;
- Ovary cancer (mortality) for women over the age of 65 has increased by 47% in African American women and 13% in Caucasian women due to genital use of talc powder;
- Breast cancer is increasing 17% due to a wide range of factors. These include: birth control pills; estrogen replacement therapy; toxic hormonal ingredients in cosmetics and personal care products; diagnostic radiation; and routine premenopausal mammography, with a cumulative breast dose exposure of up to about five rads over ten years. Reflecting these concerns, Representatives Debbie Wasserman-Schultz and Henry Waxman have introduced bills promoting educational campaigns, including teaching regular breast self examination to high school students. However, and in spite of its scientifically proven efficacy, this initiative has been strongly challenged by breast cancer prevention "experts" who remain unaware of the scientific evidence on the cancer risks of high dose radiation premenopausal mammography. Furthermore, these "experts" are unaware of the well-documented scientific evidence of avoidable causes of breast cancer, other than factors related to . . . "childbirth and breastfeeding."

It is now beyond dispute in the independent scientific community that environmental and occupational exposures to carcinogens are the primary cause of non-smoking related cancers. An October 2007 publication on environmental and occupational causes of cancer by one of us (Dr. Richard

Clapp) further emphasized that the increasing incidence of cancer is due to preventable exposures to carcinogens in the workplace and environment.

The Clapp report provides a wide range of evidence showing preventable cancers resulting from environmental exposures to formaldehyde, chlorinated organic pesticides, and organic solvents, among other substances.

The Clapp report also cites a wealth of evidence attributing the increasing incidence of lung cancers to preventable occupational exposures to asbestos, silica, chromium VI, formaldehyde, methylene chloride, benzene, and ethylene oxide.

The National Cancer Institute is the primary federal agency devoted exclusively to fighting cancer. Paradoxically, the escalating incidence of cancer over the last thirty years parallels its sharply escalating annual budget—from $690 million in 1975 to $5 billion this year. Of this a mere $131 million is allocated to NCI's mission on Prevention and Early Detection. Furthermore, President Obama has proposed a 5% increase in funding the NCI for unspecified cancer research, with a doubling to $11.5 billion over the next eight years.

However, in spite of well-documented evidence relating the escalating incidence of cancer to a wide range of avoidable carcinogenic exposures, the NCI remains "asleep at the wheel," and has stubbornly refused to devote significant resources or even attention to prevention.

The NCI has also ignored proddings from Congress and independent scientific experts to develop a comprehensive registry of carcinogens. Worse still, the NCI has misled the public by claiming that most cancers are due to unhealthy behavior, "blaming the victim," despite overwhelming evidence to the contrary.

NCI officials still claim, for instance that 94% of all cancers are due to "unhealthy behavior" such as smoking, poor nutrition, inactivity, obesity and over exposure to sunlight—and that a mere 6% are attributable to exposures to environmental and occupational exposures.

These estimates are based on those published in 1981 by the late U.K. epidemiologist Sir Richard Doll. However, from 1976 to 1999, Doll had been a closet consultant to U.K. and U.S. industries, including General Motors, Monsanto and the asbestos industry. Following revelation of these conflicts of interest, just prior to his death in 2002, Doll admitted that most cancers, other than those related to smoking and hormones, "are induced by exposure to chemicals often environmental."

Furthermore, the NCI has touted the imminent success of new cancer treatments—promises that have seldom borne out, and which have been widely questioned by the independent scientific community. For instance, in 2004, Nobel Laureate Leland Hartwell, President of the Fred Hutchinson

Cancer Control Center, warned that Congress and the public are paying NCI $4.7 billion a year, most of which is spent on "promoting ineffective drugs" for terminal disease.

As members of the independent scientific community, we welcome the Obama Administration's goal of health care reform and prevention. But while President Obama has put forward a unique cancer plan, it focuses far too much on the diagnosis and treatment of cancer, rather than on prevention. The simple truth is that the more cancer is prevented, the less there is to treat. That will also save lives and money.

Congress now has an epochal opportunity to reform our health care system and prevent diseases, particularly cancer, from occurring in the first place. By taking some simple steps, Congress should enact reforms to prevent cancer. Accordingly, we recommend that Congress enact the following specific legislative reforms to the 1971 National Cancer Act:

- Congress declares that it is the national policy of the United States to reduce carcinogenic exposures to confirmed or suspected carcinogens by at least half during the next decade.
- Congress shall create a Deputy Director for Cancer Prevention of the NCI who, in consultation with the administrators of EPA, OSHA, CPSC, FDA and other relevant regulatory agencies, shall report to Congress annually on steps needed during the next decade, under existing regulatory authority, to reduce, by at least half, exposures reasonably anticipated to reduce the prevalence of future preventable cancers.
- The Deputy Director of NCI shall meet quarterly with the administrators of EPA, OSHA, CPSC, FDA and other relevant regulatory agencies to identify opportunities to reduce exposures to carcinogens in the environment, the workplace, pharmaceuticals, and consumer products—food, household products, and cosmetics and personal care products.
- The Deputy Director's annual report shall include recommendations for changes in statutes, regulations and enforcement authority, necessary to achieve this national policy, in consultation with the administrators of the EPA, OSHA, CPSC, FDA and other relevant regulatory agencies.
- Congress shall allocate at least 40% of the NCI budget to explicit prevention related programs for FY 2011, and 50% by FY 2014.
- Congress shall mandate the annual publication of a comprehensive register of carcinogens. This will provide federal, state and local governments, as well as the public, with comprehensive information

on carcinogens in the workplace, environment, and consumer products so that necessary preventive action can be promptly undertaken.

These steps alone will not win the war against cancer, but they will be critical in redirecting a failing war on cancer that can best be described as one of the most notorious public health failures of the 20th century. Cancer prevention is a critical public policy area in which reform is long overdue.

ENDORSERS:

Nicholas A. Ashford, PhD, JD
Professor of Technology and Policy
Director, MIT Technology and Law Program
Massachusetts Institute of Technology

Richard W. Clapp, DSc, MPH
Professor Environmental Health
Boston University School of Public Health

Quentin D. Young, MD
Past President American Public Health Association
Chairman, Health and Medicine Policy Research Group, Chicago

July 17, 2009

ANOTHER REASON FOR HEALTH CARE REFORM: WINNING THE WAR ON CANCER

The cancer epidemic strikes as many as one in three Americans and takes the life of one in four. After 37 years of losing the war against cancer (a war that President Nixon originally declared in December 1971), the federal government is utterly failing to protect us from this menace. This year, 1.5 million people will be diagnosed with cancer. 562,000 people—over 1,500 every day—will die.

In a recent letter to key Congressional committees, leading representatives of the independent scientific community—those with no financial ties to polluters and the cancer drug industry—argued that the majority of non-smoking related cancers are soaring, and that this epidemic is due to preventable exposures to cancer-causing contaminants in our environment and the workplace, and ingredients in our consumer products.

The letter appeared to be instrumental in getting the Europeans to act. Citing the letter to Congress, Europe's leading environment watchdog, the Health and Environment Alliance (HEAL) last week reported that the European Commission's Communication on Cancer had "for the first time, the Commission officially acknowledges that cancer prevention should address lifestyle, occupational and environmental causes on an equal footing."

The evidence that environmental causes are the primary cause of preventable cancer is becoming overwhelming. For instance, non-Hodgkins lymphoma is preventable, but its incidence has skyrocketed by 76% in recent years due mostly to common herbicides and black hair dyes. Thyroid cancer has increased by 124% because of unnecessary exposures to ionizing radiation. Testicular cancer has increased by 50%, an increase attributable to pesticides, hormonal residues in meat, as well as hormonal ingredients in personal care and cosmetic products. Childhood leukemia and other cancers, many of which have predominantly environmental causes, are all also increasing dramatically.

Based on recent estimates by the National Institutes of Health, the total costs of cancer are $219 billion a year. The annual costs to taxpayers of diagnosis and treatment amount to $89 billion; the annual costs of premature death are conservatively estimated at $112 billion; and the annual costs due to lost productivity are conservatively estimated at $18 billion. And these are quantifiable, inflationary economic costs. The human costs are of far greater magnitude.

The connection between our losing the cancer war and the need to control costs through prevention is clear. Cancer is not only one of the most costly and sometimes fatal diseases, it is also one of the most avoidable.

Leading figures in the scientific and public health communities have joined together to petition Congress and our federal agencies to enforce the laws that are supposed to protect us from avoidable exposures to carcinogens.

But this fight is going to require a massive grass roots effort to demand that our federal government make cancer prevention a priority, and also to regulate the polluters who funnel unprecedented amounts of carcinogens in our environment, workplaces, and consumer products each day.

August 11, 2009

HOW TO FIGHT CANCER

Nobelist James Watson's August 5 New York Times Op-Ed "To Fight Cancer, Know Thy Enemy" could not be any more right. However, Watson could not be any more wrong in his belief that new "miracle drugs acting alone or in combination" are the answer, warns Dr. Samuel Epstein, chairman of the Cancer Prevention Coalition.

"The right answer is to take action to prevent cancer before it starts, he says.

Watson's belief in "miracle drugs" is echoed by claims of the National Cancer Institute (NCI) for the success of "innovative treatment" or "targeted drugs."

However, Nobelist Leland Hartwell, President of the Fred Hutchinson Cancer Control Center and leading national oncologist, warned in 2004 that "Congress and the public are now paying NCI $4.7 billion a year," most of which is spent on "promoting ineffective drugs" for terminal disease.

Furthermore, the costs of these new biotech drugs have increased over 100-fold over the last decade without any evidence supporting their effectiveness in improving survival rates.

Meanwhile, the NCI budget has escalated further to $5 billion this year, of which a mere $130 million, 2.6%, is allocated to prevention.

Reflecting concerns that cancer prevention received no attention in President Obama's Cancer Plan, a June 9 letter by Dr. Epstein and 20 other national experts on prevention was addressed to four Congressional committees: the Senate Committee on Health, Education, Labor and Pensions; the Senate Appropriations Committee; the House Committee on Energy and Commerce; and the House Appropriations Committee.

We recommended that Congress enact legislative reforms to the 1971 National Cancer Act, including a statement that it is the policy of the United States to reduce cancer-causing (carcinogenic) exposures by at least half during the next decade.

We also recommended that the NCI be responsible for the publication of a comprehensive public register of all known carcinogens in air, water, consumer products and the workplace, with annual updates as necessary.

Finally, we recommended major policy changes for the NCI. These included the appointment of a new Deputy Director for Cancer Prevention, and the allocation of at least 40% of the Institute's budget to prevention programs as from 2010.

The Obama Administration has so far been unresponsive to any of these recommendations.

March 29, 2010

FRANK CONFLICTS OF INTEREST IN THE NATIONAL CANCER INSTITUTE

In March 2010, the White House nominated Nobel Laureate Harold Varmus as Director of the National Cancer Institute (NCI).

As a key advisor to President Obama's 2008 Presidential campaign, Varmus was subsequently appointed Co-Chairman of the President's Council of Advisors on Science and Technology. He was previously President of the New York Memorial Sloan-Kettering Cancer Center.

Varmus has a distinguished track record in basic research on cancer treatment. However, as emphasized by the Cancer Prevention Coalition, this is paralleled by lack of familiarity with mounting scientific evidence on cancer prevention. Two decades ago, he claimed, "You can't do experiments to see what causes cancer—it's not an accessible problem, and not the sort of thing scientists can afford to do—everything you do can't be risky."

In 1995, Varmus, then Director of the National Institutes of Health, struck the "reasonable pricing clause," protecting against exorbitant industry profiteering from the sale of drugs, developed with tax payer money. Varmus also gave senior NCI staff free license to consult with the cancer drug industry.

In this connection, the 2008 edition of Charity Rating Guide & Watchdog Report listed Dr. Varmus with a compensation package of about $2.7 million. This is the highest compensation of over 500 major non-profit organizations ever monitored.

As a past major recipient of NCI funds for basic genetic research, Varmus warned that "reasonable pricing" clauses, protecting against exorbitant industry profiteering from drugs developed with tax-payer dollars, were driving away private industry. So he struck these from agreements between industry and the NCI. As a consequence, Varmus eliminated any price controls on cancer drugs made at the tax-payer expense.

Illustratively, using taxpayers' money, NCI paid for the research and development of Taxol, an anticancer drug, later manufactured by Bristol-Myers Squibb. Following completion of clinical trials, an extremely expensive process in itself, the public paid again for developing the drug's manufacturing process. Once completed, NCI officials gave Bristol-Myers Squibb the exclusive right to sell Taxol at an inflationary price. As investigative journalist, Joel Bleifuss, warned in a 1995 In These Times article, "Bristol-Myers Squibb sells Taxol to the public for $4.87 per milligram, which is more than 20 times what it costs to produce." Taxol has been a blockbuster for Bristol-Myers, posting sales of over $3 billion since its approval in 1992, and accounting for about 40 percent of the company's sales.

Taxol was not the only drug involved in such funding practices. Bristol-Myers Squibb now sells nearly one-third of the approximately thirty-five cancer drugs currently available, often with highly inflated profits, and often developed with taxpayer funds. In 1995, Varmus, a past major recipient of NCI funds for basic genetic research, decided that "reasonable pricing" clauses, protecting against profiteering from drugs developed with taxpayer dollars, were driving away private industry. So he struck these from pricing clauses.

Taxol was not an isolated example. Taxpayers have funded NCI's research and development for over two-thirds of all cancer drugs now on the market. In a surprisingly frank admission, Samuel Broder, NCI Director from 1989 to 1995, stated the obvious: "The NCI has become what amounts to a government pharmaceutical company." Nobel Laureate Leland Hartwell, President of the Fred Hutchinson Cancer Research Center, endorsed Broder's criticism. He further stressed that most resources for cancer research are spent on "promoting ineffective drugs" for terminal disease. In this connection, Memorial Sloan-Kettering's Leonard Saltz estimated that the price for new biotech drugs "has increased 500-fold in the last decade." Furthermore, the U.S. spends five times more than the U.K. on cancer chemotherapy per patient, although survival rates are similar.

As an expert in cancer treatment, Varmus appears unaware that almost 700 carcinogens, to some of which the public is periodically or regularly exposed, have been identified by independent scientists. He also seems to be unaware that the more cancer is prevented the less there is to treat.

On June 15, 2009, a letter to Congressional leaders urging drastic reform of the Obama Cancer Plan to mandate prevention, besides urging the annual publication of a public registry of carcinogens, was released by the five scientists listed below. This letter also listed seven cancers, summarized their avoidable causes, and their increasing incidence since 1975, based on 2005 NCI data:

- Malignant melanoma (mortality) of the skin in adults has increased by 168% due to the use of sunscreens in childhood that fail to block long wave ultraviolet light;
- Thyroid cancer has increased by 124% due in large part to ionizing radiation;
- Non-Hodgkin's lymphoma has increased by 76% due mostly to phenoxy herbicides; and phenylenediamine hair dyes;
- Testicular cancer has increased by 49% due to pesticides; hormonal ingredients in cosmetics and personal care products; and estrogen residues in meat;

- Childhood leukemia has increased by 55% due to ionizing radiation; domestic pesticides; nitrite preservatives in meats, particularly hot dogs; and parental exposures to occupational carcinogens;
- Ovary cancer (mortality) for women over the age of 65 has increased by 47% in African American women and 13% in Caucasian women due to genital use of talc powder;
- Breast cancer has increased by 17% due to a wide range of factors. These include: birth control pills; toxic hormonal ingredients in cosmetics and personal care products; diagnostic radiation; and routine premenopausal mammography, with a cumulative breast dose exposure of up to about five rads over ten years.

However, and as an expert in cancer treatment, Varmus was unlikely to be aware of such scientific evidence, which was not widely recognized until relatively recently.

Based on recent estimates by the National Institutes of Health, the total costs of cancer are about $219 billion each year. The annual costs to taxpayers of diagnosis and treatment amounts to $89 billion; the annual costs of premature death are conservatively estimated at $112 billion; and the annual costs due to loss of productivity are conservatively estimated at $18 billion. The human costs surely are of far greater magnitude. Much of these costs could be saved by cancer prevention.

These concerns regarding Dr. Varmus have been recognized and endorsed by the following leading national experts on cancer prevention:

Rosalie Bertell, PhD
Regent, International Physicians for Humanitarian Medicine

Richard Clapp, DSc, MPH
Professor, Boston University School of Public Health

Janette D. Sherman, MD
New York Academy of Science, 2009

Quentin D. Young, MD
Chairman, Health and Medicine Policy Research Group

May 4, 2010

CANCER PREVENTION COALITION URGED SUPPORT OF THE SAFE CHEMICALS ACT

The Cancer Prevention Coalition encouraged people to support the Safe Chemicals Act of 2010, introduced by Senator Frank Lautenberg (D-NJ) on April 15 this year. This amends the 1976 Toxic Substances Control Act by requiring manufacturers to prove the safety of chemicals before they are marketed. Of particular concern are carcinogens, to which the public remains dangerously exposed and uninformed.

In 1971, President Richard Nixon declared the national "war against cancer," and the National Cancer Act was passed. This charged the National Cancer Institute (NCI) "to disseminate cancer information to the public."

The 1971 Act also authorized the President to appoint the director of NCI and control its budget, thus bypassing the scientific and budgetary authority of the director of 26 other National Institutes of Health (NIH).

As a result of this anomaly, NCI's current $5.3 billion budget, 17% that of the entire NIH, remains beyond control of NIH's director.

This special status of the NCI was challenged in 2003 by the National Academy of Sciences, at hearings of the House Energy and Commerce, and also by the Senate Health, Education, Labor and Pensions Committees.

Furthermore, contrary to the specific requirements of the 1971 Act, the NCI has still failed to "disseminate cancer information to the public," and to warn the public of a wide range of avoidable causes of cancer.

The 1988 amendments to the National Cancer Program called for "an expanded and identified research program for the prevention of cancer caused by occupational or environmental exposure to carcinogens." However, these amendments have been and remain ignored by the NCI.

For over four decades, NCI policies have been and remain fixated on damage control—screening, diagnosis, treatment and related research. Meanwhile priorities for prevention, from avoidable exposures to carcinogens in air, water, consumer products, and the workplace have remained minimal.

To be sure, smoking remains the best-known and single largest cause of cancer, particularly lung cancer. However, while lung cancer incidence rates in men have declined by 20% over the past three decades, those in women have increased by 111%. But more importantly, non-smoking cancers—due to known chemical and physical carcinogens—have increased substantially since 1975.

Some of the more startling realities in the failure to prevent cancer are illustrated by their soaring increases. Examples include:

Malignant melanoma of the skin in adults has increased by 168% due to the use of sunscreens in childhood that fail to block long wave ultraviolet light;

Thyroid cancer has increased by 124% due in large part to ionizing radiation;

Non-Hodgkin's lymphoma has increased 76% due mostly to phenoxy herbicides; and phenylenediamine hair dyes;

Testicular cancer has increased by 49% due to pesticides; hormonal ingredients in cosmetics and personal care products; and estrogen residues in meat;

Childhood leukemia has increased by 55% due to ionizing radiation; domestic pesticides; nitrite preservatives in meats, particularly hot dogs; and parental exposures to occupational carcinogens;

Ovary cancer (mortality) for women over the age of 65 has increased by 47% in African American women and 13% in Caucasian women due to genital use of talc powder;

Breast cancer has increased 17% due to a wide range of factors. These include: birth control pills; estrogen replacement therapy; toxic hormonal ingredients in cosmetics and personal care products; diagnostic radiation; and routine premenopausal mammography, with a cumulative breast dose exposure of up to about five rads over ten years. Reflecting these concerns, Representatives Debbie Wasserman-Schultz and Henry Waxman have introduced bills promoting educational campaigns, including teaching regular breast self examination to high school students.

Paradoxically the escalating incidence of cancer over the last thirty years parallels its sharply escalating annual budget, from $690 million in 1975 to $5.2 billion this year. Of this, a mere $314 million (6%) is claimed to be allocated to NCI's mission on "Cancer Prevention and Control."

However, in spite of well-documented evidence relating the escalating incidence of cancer to a wide range of avoidable carcinogenic exposures, the NCI remains "asleep at the wheel," and has recklessly refused to devote significant resources to prevention.

The NCI has also ignored proddings from Congress and independent scientific experts to develop a comprehensive registry of carcinogens. Worse still, the NCI has misled the public by claiming that most cancers are due to "unhealthy behavior," blaming the victim, despite overwhelming evidence to the contrary.

For instance, the NCI still claimed that 94% of all cancers are due to "unhealthy behavior," such as smoking, poor nutrition, inactivity, obesity and over exposure to sunlight, while a mere 6% are attributable to environmental and occupational exposures.

These estimates are based on those published in 1981 by the late U.K. epidemiologist Richard Doll. However, from 1976 to 1999, Doll had been a closet consultant to U.K. and U.S. industries, including General Motors, Monsanto and the asbestos industry. Following revelation of these conflicts of interest, just prior to his death in 2002, Doll admitted that most cancers, other than those related to smoking and hormones, "are induced by exposure to chemicals often environmental."

Furthermore the NCI has touted the imminent success of new cancer treatments, but says these promises have seldom borne out, and have been widely questioned by the independent scientific community.

For instance, Nobel Laureate Leland Hartwell, President of the Fred Hutchinson Cancer Control Center, warned in 2004 that Congress and the public are paying NCI $4.7 billion a year, most of which is spent on "promoting ineffective drugs" for terminal disease.

Based on recent estimates by the National Institutes of Health, the total costs of cancer have now reached $228 billion a year. The annual costs to taxpayers of diagnosis and treatment amount to $93 billion; the annual costs of premature death are conservatively estimated at $116 billion; and the annual costs due to lost productivity are conservatively estimated at $19 billion. These are quantifiable and inflationary economic costs. The human costs surely are of far greater magnitude.

January 10, 2011

UNRECOGNIZED DANGERS OF FORMALDEHYDE

A December 10, 2010 a two page article in *The New York Times*, "When Wrinkle-Free Clothing Also Means Formaldehyde Fumes," stated that "formaldehyde is commonly found in a broad range of consumer products." These include sheets, pillow cases and drapes, besides "personal care products like shampoos, lotions and eye shadows." It was stated in this article that "most of the 180 items tested, largely clothes and bed linens, had low or undetectable levels of formaldehyde that met voluntary industry guidelines." Most consumers will probably never have a problem with exposure to formaldehyde," since such low levels "are not likely to irritate most people," other than those wearing wrinkle-resistant clothing. "The U.S. does not regulate formaldehyde levels in clothing. Nor does any government agency require manufacturers to disclose the use of this chemical on labels."

On March 5, 2008, Senators Bob Casey, Sherrod Brown and Mary Landrieu introduced an amendment to the Consumer Product Safety Commission (CPSC) reform bill "that would help protect Americans from dangerous levels of formaldehyde in textiles including clothing." The Senators referred to a 1997 CPSC report on formaldehyde, which admitted that "it causes cancer in tests on laboratory animals, and may cause cancer in humans." Accordingly, the senators requested the CPSC to "regulate and test formaldehyde in textiles and protect consumers from this poison."

In August 2010, a Government Accountability Office (GAO) report warned that "a small proportion of the U.S. population does have allergic reactions to formaldehyde resins on their clothes." However, the GAO made no recommendations for any regulatory action.

It is surprising that many people are unaware of the longstanding scientific evidence on the carcinogenicity of formaldehyde. However, this had been detailed in five National Toxicology Program Reports on Carcinogens from 1981 to 2004. These classified formaldehyde as "reasonably anticipated to be a human carcinogen," based on limited evidence of carcinogenicity in humans, and sufficient evidence in experimental animals. This evidence was confirmed in a series of reports by the prestigious International Agency for Research on Cancer (IARC). Its 2006 and 2010 reports explicitly warn that formaldehyde is "a known cause of leukemia in experimental animals—and nasal cancer" in humans.

"Strong" evidence of the nasal cancer risk was also cited in the May 2010 President's Cancer Panel report, "Environmental Cancer Risk: What Can We Do Now?" Nevertheless, and in spite of this explicit evidence, a September

2010 Government Accountability Office report attempted to trivialize the cancer risks of formaldehyde on the alleged grounds that exposure levels are low or "non-detectable."

Of further concern, occupational exposure to formaldehyde has been associated with breast cancer deaths in a 1995 National Cancer Institute report, while environmental exposure has been associated with an increased incidence of breast cancer in a 2005 University of Texas report.

None of the dermatologists quoted in *The New York Times* appear aware of long-standing evidence that most cosmetics and personal care products, commonly used daily by most women, besides on their infants and children, and to a lesser extent men, contain up to eight ingredients which are precursors of formaldehyde. These include diazolidinyl urea, metheneamine and quaterniums, each of which readily breaks down on the skin to release formaldehyde. This is then readily absorbed through the skin, and poses unknowing risks of cancer to the majority of the U.S. population.

AMERICAN CANCER SOCIETY

More Interested in Accumulating Wealth Than Saving Lives

ENDORSED BY
Congressman John Conyers, Jr.
United States Representative (MI-14)
Second most senior member of the House
Chairman, the House Judiciary Committee

Quentin D. Young, MD
Chairman, Health and Medicine Policy Research Group
Illinois Public Health Advocate
Past President, American Public Health Association

ORGANIZATION

The American Cancer Society (ACS) Inc. consists of a National Home Office with thirteen chartered divisions throughout the United States and a presence in most communities.

Fact Sheet

"The American Cancer Society is a nationwide community-based voluntary health organization dedicated to eliminating cancer as a major health problem by preventing cancer, saving lives, and diminishing suffering from cancer through research, education, advocacy, and service. With more than two million volunteers nationwide, the American Cancer Society is one of the oldest and largest voluntary health agencies in the United States."

The National Home Office is responsible for the overall planning and coordination of the Society's programs for cancer information delivery, cancer control and prevention, advocacy, resource development, and patient services. The national office also provides technical support and materials to divisions and local offices and administers the intramural and extramural research programs. The National Board of Directors includes representatives for the divisions and the general public.

The Divisions

The Society's thirteen divisions are governed by boards of directors composed of medical and lay volunteers throughout the United States and Puerto Rico. The divisions are responsible for program delivery service in their regions.

Local Offices

More than 3,400 local offices nationwide are organized to deliver information on cancer prevention and early detection and patient service programs at the community level.

Volunteers

More than two million volunteers carry out the Society's mission of eliminating cancer and improving quality of life for those facing the disease. These volunteers donate their time and talents to educate the public about early detection and prevention; advocate for responsible cancer legislation in local, state, and federal governments; and serve cancer patients and their families as they manage their cancer experience

HISTORY

The ACS, then known as the American Society for the Control of Cancer (ASCC), was founded in 1913 in New York City by fifteen prominent MDs, largely oncologists. It was incorporated in 1922 by a small group of wealthy businessmen.

In 1936, the ASCC created a legion of 15,000 volunteers, the Women's Field Army, to wage war on cancer and raise money for this purpose. By 1938, the army had recruited about 150,000 volunteers and become one of the nation's leading voluntary health organizations.

In 1945, the ASCC was reorganized and renamed the American Cancer Society (ACS). Within one year, $4 million had been raised, $1 million of which was used to establish a cancer research program. Shortly afterward, the ACS began a "public education campaign," warning of "Cancer's Danger Signals." These included: a sore that does not heal; a change in bowel habits; and faulty lifestyle, such as poor diet. However, there was no consideration whatsoever of any other then well-known avoidable causes of cancer.

In 1971, the ACS aggressively campaigned President Nixon to declare the War on Cancer, claiming that this could be won, given increased funding for the National Cancer Institute (NCI). President Nixon responded by increasing its funding by $200,000. This was in excess of the funding that it then received as one of thirty other National Institutes of Health. In so doing, President Nixon effectively created an independent status for the NCI.

The ACS and NCI have long continued to devote virtually exclusive priority to research on diagnosis and treatment of cancer, with indifference to prevention, other than faulty personal lifestyle, commonly known as blame the victim, to the exclusion of a very wide range of then well-documented avoidable causes of cancer. The long-standing exclusionary emphasis of the ACS and to a lesser extent the NCI, on the "blame the victim" cause of cancer was based on the claims of Sir Richard Doll, a closet industry consultant. The

NCI's current budget of about $5.2 until very recently remains largely directed to these very limited objectives. Not surprisingly, the incidence of cancer over the past decades has escalated, approximately parallel to its increased funding.

According to James Bennett, a recognized authority on charitable organizations, in 1988 the ACS held a fund balance of over $400 million with about $69 million of holdings in land, building, and equipment. However, the ACS spent only $90 million, 26% of its budget, on medical research and programs. The rest covered operating expenses, including about 60% for generous salaries, pensions, executive benefits, and overhead. By 1989, the cash reserves of the ACS were more than $700 million.

In 1991, believing it was contributing to fighting cancer, the public gave nearly $350 million to the ACS. Most of this money came from donations averaging $3,500, besides high-profile fund-raising campaigns, such as the springtime daffodil sale and the May relay races. However, over subsequent decades, an increasing proportion of the ACS budget has come from large corporations, including the pharmaceutical, cancer drug, telecommunications, and entertainment industries.

In 1992, the American Cancer Society Foundation was created to allow the ACS to solicit contributions of more than $100,000. A close look at the heavy hitters on the foundation's board made it clear what conflicts of interests were at play and from where the foundation expected its big contributions. The foundation's board of trustees included corporate executives from the pharmaceutical, investment, banking, and media industries. These included as follows:

- David R. Bethune, president of Lederle Laboratories, a multinational pharmaceutical company and a division of American Cyanamid Company. Bethune was also vice president of American Cyanamid, which made chemical fertilizers and herbicides while transforming itself into a full-fledged pharmaceutical company. In 1988, American Cyanamid introduced Novatrone, an anticancer drug, and subsequently announced that it would buy a majority of shares of Immunex, a cancer drug industry.

- Gordon Binder, CEO of Amgen, the world's foremost biotechnology company, with over $1 billion in product sales in 1992. Amgen's success rested almost exclusively on one product, Neupogen, administered to chemotherapy patients to stimulate production of their white blood cells.

- Multimillionaire Irwin Beck, whose father, William Henry Beck, founded Beck's Stores, the nation's largest family-owned retail chain, which brought in revenues of $1.7 billion in 1993.

- Diane Disney Miller, daughter of the conservative multimillionaire Walt Disney, and wife of Ron Miller, former president of the Walt Disney Company from 1980 to 1984.
- George Dessert, famous in media circles for his former role as censor on family values during the 1970s and 1980s, as CEO of CBS and, subsequently, ACS board chairman.
- Alan Gevertzen, 1992 chairman of Boeing, the world's then number one commercial aircraft maker, with net sales of $30 billion.
- Sumner M. Redstone, chairman of Viacom International Inc., a broadcasting, telecommunications, entertainment, and cable television corporation.

The ACS fund-raising was very successful. A million here, a million there, much of it coming from the very industries instrumental in shaping ACS policy or profiting from it.

A 1992 article in the *Wall Street Journal*, by Thomas DiLorenzo, professor of economics at Loyola College and veteran investigator of nonprofit organizations, revealed that the Texas affiliate of the ACS owned more than $11 million of assets in land and real estate, more than 56 vehicles, including 11 Ford Crown Victorias for senior executives, and 45 other cars assigned to staff members. ACS chapters in Arizona, California, and Missouri spent only 10% of their funds on direct community services. Thus for every $1 spent on direct services, approximately $6.40 was spent on compensation and overhead. In all ten states, salaries and fringe benefits were, by far, the largest single budget items, a surprising fact in light of the characterization of the appeals, which stressed an urgent and critical need for donations to provide cancer services.

In 1993, the *Chronicle of Philanthropy* published a statement that the ACS was "more interested in accumulating wealth than in saving lives." Fund-raising appeals routinely stated that the ACS needed more funds to support its cancer programs, all the while holding more than $750 million in cash and real estate assets.

Nationally, only 16% or less of all money raised was spent on direct services to cancer victims, like driving cancer patients from the hospital after chemotherapy and providing pain medication.

Most of the funds raised by the ACS have gone and still go to pay overhead, salaries, fringe benefits, and travel expenses of its national executives in Atlanta. They also go to pay chief executive officers, who earn six-figure salaries in several states, and the hundreds of other employees who work out of some 3,000 regional offices nationwide. The typical ACS affiliate, which helps raise the money for the national office, spent more than 52% of its budget on salaries, pensions, fringe benefits, and overhead for its own employees. Salaries and overhead of most ACS affiliates also exceeded 50% although most direct community services were handled by unpaid volunteers. DiLorenzo summed up his 1992 findings by emphasizing the ACS hoarding of funds.

> If current needs are not being met because of insufficient funds, as fund-raising appeals suggest, why is so much cash being hoarded? Most contributors believe their donations are being used to fight cancer, not to accumulate financial reserves. More progress in the war against cancer would be made if they would divest some of their real estate holding and use the proceeds—as well as a portion of their cash reserves—to provide more cancer services.

Aside from high salaries and overhead, most of what was left of the ACS budget has gone to research on profitable patented cancer drugs.

As of 1998, the ACS budget was $380 million, with cash reserves approaching $1 billion. Yet its aggressive fund-raising campaign continued, and still continues, to plead poverty and lament the lack of available money for cancer research. Meanwhile, efforts to prevent cancer by phasing out avoidable exposures to environmental and occupational carcinogens remained ignored. The ACS also remained silent about its intricate relationships with the wealthy cancer drug, chemical, and other industries.

A March 30, 1998, Associated Press release shed unexpected light on questionable ACS expenditures on lobbying. National vice president for federal and state governmental relations Linda Hay Crawford admitted that over the last year, the Society used ten of its own senior employees on direct lobbying. For legal and other help, it hired the lobbying firm of Hogan & Hartson, whose roster included former House Minority Leader Robert H. Michel (R-IL). The lobbying also included $30,000 donations to Democratic and Republican governors' associations. "We wanted to look like players and be players," explained Crawford. This practice, however, had been sharply challenged. An Associated Press release quoted the national Charities Information Bureau as then stating it "does not know of any other charity that makes contributions to political parties."

Not surprisingly, tax experts warned that these contributions could be illegal as charities are not allowed to make political donations. Marcus Owens, director of the IRS Exempt Organization Division, also warned that "the bottom line is campaign contributions will jeopardize a charity's tax exempt status." This warning still remains unheeded.

Marching in lockstep with the NCI in its war on cancer is the ACS's ministry of information. With powerful media control and public relations resources, the ACS was and still remains the tail that wags the dog of NCI's policies and priorities. These reflected a virtually exclusive "blame the victim" philosophy and emphasized faulty lifestyle rather than unknowing and avoidable exposures to workplace and environmental and other carcinogens. Giant corporations—which profited handsomely while they polluted air, water, the workplace, and food with a wide range of carcinogens—remain greatly comforted by the silence of the ACS. This silence reflected a complex of mind-sets fixated on diagnosis, treatment, and basic genetic research, together with ignorance, indifference, and even hostility to prevention. These mind-sets are also coupled with major conflicts of interest.

Indeed, despite promises to the public to do everything to "wipe out cancer in your lifetime," the ACS has failed to make its voice heard in Congress and the regulatory arena. Instead, the ACS has consistently rejected or ignored opportunities and requests from Congress, regulatory agencies, unions, and environmental and consumer organizations to provide scientific evidence critical to efforts to legislate and occupational, environmental, and personal product carcinogens.

The War Against Cancer

The launching of President Nixon's 1971 war against cancer provided the ACS with a well-exploited opportunity to pursue it own myopic and self-interested agenda.

ACS conflicts of interest are extensive and still largely unrecognized by the public. Meanwhile, the ACS continues to ignore a wide range of industrial carcinogens in water, air, food, the workplace, and in mainstream household, cosmetics, and personal care products.

ACS strategies remain based on two myths: First that there has been dramatic progress in the treatment and cure of cancer, and second, that any increase in the incidence and mortality of cancer is due to aging of the population and smoking while denying any significant role for involuntary exposures to industrial and other carcinogens.

As the world's largest nonreligious charity, with powerful allies in the private and public sectors, ACS policies and priorities remain unchanged. Despite periodic protest, threats of boycotts, and questions on its finances, the ACS leadership responds with powerful public relations campaigns reflecting denial and manipulated information while pillorying its opponents with scientific McCarthyism.

The verdict is unassailable. The ACS bears a major decades-long responsibility for losing the winnable war against cancer. Reforming the ACS is, in principle, relatively easy and directly achievable. Boycott the ACS. Instead, give your charitable contributions to public interest and environmental groups involved in cancer prevention. Such a boycott is well overdue and will send the only message this charity can no longer ignore.

FRANK CONFLICTS
OF INTEREST

Of the members of the ACS board, about half are clinicians, oncologists, surgeons, radiologists, and basic molecular scientists, mostly with close ties to the NCI. Many board members and their institutional colleagues apply for and obtain funding from both the ACS and the NCI. Substantial NCI funds also go to ACS directors who sit on key NCI committees. Although the ACS asks board members to leave the room when the rest of the board discusses their funding proposals, this is just a token formality. In this private club, easy access to funding is one of the perks and the board routinely rubber-stamps approvals. A significant amount of ACS research funding goes to this extended membership. Frank conflicts of interest are evident in many ACS priorities. These include their policies on mammography, the National Breast Cancer Awareness campaign, and the pesticide and cancer drug industries. These conflicts even extend to the privatization of national cancer policy.

Mammography

The ACS has close connections to the mammography industry. As detailed in the author's 1998 *The Politics of Cancer Revisited*, five radiologists have served as ACS presidents, and in its every move, the ACS reflects the interests of the major manufacturers of mammogram machines and films. These include Siemens, DuPont, General Electric, Eastman Kodak, and Piker. In fact, if every woman followed ACS and NCI mammography guidelines, the annual revenue to health care facilities would be a staggering $5 billion.

ACS promotion continues to lure women of all ages into mammography centers, leading them to believe that mammography is their best hope against breast cancer. A leading Massachusetts newspaper featured a photograph of two women in their twenties in an ACS advertisement that promised early detection results in a cure "nearly 100 percent of the time." An ACS communications director, questioned by journalist Kate Dempsey, responded in an article published by the Massachusetts Women's Community's journal *Cancer*: "The ad isn't based on a study. When you make an advertisement, you just say what you can to get women in the door. You exaggerate a point. Mammography today is a lucrative [and] highly competitive business."

In addition, the mammography industry conducts research for the ACS and its grantees, serves on advisory boards, and donates considerable funs. DuPont is a substantial backer of the ACS Breast Health Awareness Program; sponsors television shows and other media productions touting mammography; produces advertising, promotional, and educational literature and films for hospitals, clinics, medical organizations, and doctors; and lobbies Congress for legislation promoting availability of mammography services. In virtually all of these important actions, the ACS remains strongly linked with the mammography industry while ignoring the development of viable alternatives to mammography, particularly breast self-examination.

The ACS exposes premenopausal women to radiation hazards from mammography with little or no evidence of benefits. The ACS also fails to tell them that their breasts will change so much over time that the "baseline" images have little or no future relevance. This is truly an American Cancer Society crusade. But against whom, or rather, for whom?

National Breast Cancer Awareness Month

The highly publicized National Breast Cancer Awareness Month campaign further illustrates these institutionalized conflicts of interest. Every October, ACS and NCI representatives help sponsor promotional events, hold interviews, and stress the need for mammography. The flagship of this month-long series of events is the October 15 National Mammography Day.

Conspicuously absent from the widely promoted National Breast Cancer Awareness Month is any information on environmental and other avoidable causes of breast cancer. This is no accident. Zeneca Pharmaceuticals—a spin-off of Imperial Chemical Industries—is one of the world's largest manufacturers of chlorinated and other industrial chemicals, including those incriminated as causes of breast cancer. Zeneca has also been the sole multimillion-dollar funder of the National Breast Cancer Awareness Month since its inception in 1984 besides the sole manufacturer of Tamoxifen, the world's top-selling anticancer and breast cancer prevention drug, with $400 million in annual sales. Furthermore, Zeneca recently assumed direct management of eleven cancer centers in U.S. hospitals. Zeneca owns a 50% stake in these centers known collectively as Salick Health Care.

The link between the ACS, NCI, and Zeneca is especially strong when it comes to Tamoxifen. The ACS and NCI continue to aggressively promote the Tamoxifen, which is the cornerstone of its minimal prevention program. On March 7, 1997, the NCI Press Office released a four-page statement "For Response to Inquiries on Breast Cancer." The brief section on prevention reads:

> Researchers are looking for a way to prevent breast cancer in women at high risk...A large study [is underway] to see if the drug Tamoxifen will reduce cancer risk in women age 60 or older and in women 35 to 59 who have a pattern of risk factors for breast cancer. This study is also a model for future studies of cancer prevention. Studies of diet and nutrition could also lead to preventive strategies.

Since Zeneca influences every leaflet, poster, publication, and commercial of the National Breast Cancer Awareness Month, it is no wonder that such information and publications made no mention of carcinogenic industrial chemicals and their relation to breast cancer. Imperial Chemical Industries, Zeneca's parent company, profits by manufacturing breast cancer-causing chemicals. Zeneca profits from treatment of breast cancer and hopes to profit still more from the prospects of large-scale national use of Tamoxifen for breast cancer prevention. National Breast Cancer Awareness Month is a masterful public relations coup for Zeneca, providing the company with valuable goodwill besides money from millions of American women.

The Pesticide Industry

Just how inbred is the relation between the ACS and the chemical industry became clear in the spring of 1993 to Marty Koughan, a public TV producer. Koughan was then about to broadcast a documentary on the dangers of pesticides to children for the Public Broadcasting Service's hour-long show, *Frontline*. Koughan's investigation relied heavily on the June 1993 National Academy of Sciences groundbreaking report titled "Pesticides in the Diet of Children." This report declared the nation's food supply "inadequately protected" from cancer-causing pesticides and a significant threat to the health of children.

An earlier report, "Intolerable Risk: Pesticides in Our Children's Food," by the Natural Resources Defense Council in 1989, had also given pesticide manufacturers failing marks. The report was released in high-profile testimony to Congress by movie actress Meryl Streep. A mother of young children, Streep explained to a packed House chamber the report's findings, namely, that children were most at risk from cancer-causing pesticides in food as they consume a disproportionate amount of fruits, fruit juices, and vegetables relative to their size. However, shortly before Koughan's program was due to air, a draft of the script was mysteriously leaked to Porter Novelli, a powerful public relations firm for produce growers and the agrichemical industry. In true Washington fashion, Porter Novelli played both sides of the fence, representing both government agencies and the industries they regulated. Its 1993 client list included Ciba-Geigy, DuPont, Monsanto, Burroughs Wellcome, American Petroleum Institute, Bristol-Myers Squibb, Hoffman-LaRoche, Hoechst Celanese, Hoechst Roussel Pharmaceutical, Janssen Pharmaceutical, Johnson & Johnson, the Center for Produce Quality, as well as the U.S. Department of Agriculture and the NCI besides other National Institutes of Health.

Porter Novelli first crafted a rebuttal to help quell public fears about pesticide-contaminated food. Next, Porter Novelli called up another client, the American Cancer Society for whom Porter Novelli had done pro bono work for years. The rebuttal that Porter Novelli had just sent off to its industry clients was faxed to ACS Atlanta headquarters. It was then circulated by e-mail on March 22, 1993, virtually verbatim from the memo Porter Novelli had crafted as a backgrounder for three thousand regional ACS offices to help field calls from the public after the show aired.

"The program makes unfounded suggestions . . . that pesticide residue in food may be at hazardous levels," the ACS memo read. "Its use of 'cancer cluster' leukemia case reports and non-specific community illnesses as alleged evidence of pesticide effects in people is unfortunate. We know of no community cancer cases and none in which pesticide use was confirmed as the cause."

This bold, unabashed defense of the pesticide industry, crafted by Porter Novelli, was then rehashed a third time, this time by the right-wing group, Accuracy in Media (AIM). AIM's newsletter gleefully published quotes from the ACS memo in an article with the banner headline: "Junk Science on PBS." The article opened with "Can we afford the Public Broadcasting Service?" and then went on to disparage Koughan's documentary on pesticides and children. "In Our Children's Food . . . exemplified what the media have done to produce these 'popular panics' and the enormously costly waste [at PBS] cited by the *New York Times*."

When Koughan saw the AIM article he was initially outraged that the ACS was being used to defend the pesticide industry. "At first, I assumed complete ignorance on the part of the ACS," said Koughan. But after repeatedly trying, without success, to get the national office to rebut the AIM article, Koughan began to see what was really going on. "When I realized that Porter Novelli represented five agrichemical companies, and that the ACS had been its client for years, it became obvious that the ACS had not been fooled at all," said Koughan. "They were willing partners in the deception, and were in fact doing a favor for a friend—by flaking for the agrichemical industry."

Charles Benbrook, former director of the National Academy of Sciences Board of Agriculture, charged that the role of the ACS as a source of information for the media was "unconscionable." Investigative reporter Sheila Kaplan, in a 1993 *Legal Times* article, went further: "What they did was clearly and unequivocally over the line, and constitutes a major conflict of interest."

The Cancer Drug Industry

The intimate association between the ACS and the cancer drug industry, with annual sales of over $12 billion, is further illustrated by the unbridled aggression which the ACS has directed at its critics.

Just as Senator Joseph McCarthy had his blacklist of suspected communists and Richard Nixon his environmental activist enemies list, so too the ACS maintains a Committee on Unproven Methods of Cancer Management, which periodically reviews unorthodox or alternative therapies. This committee is comprised of volunteer health care professionals, carefully selected proponents of orthodox, expensive, and usually toxic drugs patented by major pharmaceutical companies, and opponents of alternative or unproven therapies that are generally cheap, nonpatentable, and minimally toxic.

Periodically, the committee updates its statements on unproven methods, which are then widely disseminated to clinicians, cheerleader science writers, and the public. Once a clinician or oncologist becomes associated with unproven methods, he or she is blackballed by the cancer establishment. Funding for the accused quack becomes inaccessible, followed by systematic harassment.

The highly biased ACS witch-hunts against alternative practitioners is in striking contrast to its extravagant and uncritical endorsement of conventional toxic chemotherapy. This despite the absence of any objective evidence of improved survival rates or reduced mortality following chemotherapy for all but some relatively rare cancers.

In response to pressure from People against Cancer, a grassroots group of cancer patients disillusioned with conventional cancer therapy, in 1986, some forty members of Congress requested the Office of Technology Assessment (OTA), a congressional think tank, to evaluate available information on alternative innovative therapies. While initially resistant, OTA eventually published a September 1990 report that identified some two hundred promising studies on alternative therapies. OTA concluded that the NCI had "mandated responsibility to pursue this information and facilitate examination of widely used 'unconventional cancer treatments' for therapeutic potential."

Yet the ACS and NCI remained resistant, if not frankly hostile, to OTA's recommendations. In the January 1991 issue of its *Cancer Journal for Clinicians*, the ACS referred to the Hoxsey therapy, a nontoxic combination of herb extracts developed in the 1940s by populist Harry Hoxsey, as a "worthless tonic for cancer." However, a detailed critique of Hoxsey's treatment by Dr. Patricia Spain Ward, a leading contributor to the OTA report, concluded just the opposite: "More recent literature leaves no doubt that Hoxsey's formula does indeed contain many plant substances of marked therapeutic activity."

Nor is this the first time that the Society's charges of quackery have been called into question or discredited. A growing number of other innovative therapies originally attacked by the ACS have recently found less disfavor and even acceptance. These include hyperthermia, tumor necrosis factor (originally called Coley's toxin), hydrazine sulfate, and Burzynski's antineoplastons. Well over one hundred promising alternative nonpatented and nontoxic therapies have been identified. Clearly, such treatments merit clinical testing and evaluation by the NCI using similar statistical techniques and criteria as established for conventional chemotherapy. However, while the FDA has approved approximately forty patented drugs for cancer treatment, it has still not approved a single nonpatented alternative drug.

Subsequent events have further isolated the ACS in its fixation on "orthodox treatments." Bypassing the ACS and NCI, in June 1992, the National Institutes of Health opened a new Office of Alternative Medicine for the investigation of unconventional treatment of cancer and other diseases. Leading proponents of conventional therapy were invited to participate. The ACS refused. The NCI grudgingly and nominally participated while actively attacking alternative therapy with its widely circulated *Cancer Information Services*. Meanwhile, the NCI's police partner, the FDA, used its enforcement authority against distributors and practitioners of innovative and nontoxic therapies.

In an interesting development, the Washington, D.C., Center for Mind-Body Medicine, held a two-day conference on Comprehensive Cancer Care Integrating Complementary and Alternative Medicine. According to Dr. James Gordon, president of the center and chair of the Program Advisory Council of the NIH Office of Alternative Medicine, the object of the conference was to bring together practitioners of mainstream and alternative medicine, together with cancer patients and high-ranking officials of the ACS and NCI. Dr. Gordon warned alternative practitioners that "they're going to need to get more rigorous with their work—to be accepted by the mainstream community." However, no such warning was directed at the highly questionable claims of the NCI and ACS for the efficacy of conventional cancer chemotherapy. As significantly, criticism of the establishment's minimalistic priority for cancer prevention was effectively discouraged.

Privatization of National Cancer Policy

In February 2002, Senator Dianne Feinstein introduced the National Cancer Act of 2002. Cosponsored by thirty bipartisan senators, including Majority Leader Tom Daschle and Hillary Clinton, the bill was a radically different version of President Nixon's 1971 Act that launched the National Cancer Program. The bill added $1.4 billion to the $4.6 billion 2003 budget authorized by President Bush, extra funds coming from the new federal cigarette tax increase, and a further 50% annual increase to 2007, reaching a grand total of $14 billion. Feinstein said her goal was to "form our new battle plan to fight cancer." The legislation was referred to the Committee on Health, Education, Labor, and Pensions, then chaired by Senator Judd Gregg.

This bill established a national network of twenty "translation" centers to combine basic and clinical research and to commercialize promising findings. It also mandated insurance coverage for cancer screening, smoking cessation, genetic testing, and quality care standards while making no reference to prevention.

Regrettably, this well-intentioned bill surrendered the National Cancer Program to special interests. The legislation was strongly criticized by survivor coalitions, headed by the Cancer Leadership Council, and the American Society for Clinical Oncology. Of major concern, the bill displaced control of cancer policy from the public to the private sector, the federal NCI to the nonprofit ACS, raising concerns on conflicts of interest and special interests. Dr. John Durant, executive president of the American Society of Clinical Oncology (ASCO), awarded the Society's 2002 Presidential U.S. Cancer Fighter of the Year, charged, "It has always seemed to me that this was an issue of control by the ACS over the cancer agenda. They are protecting their own fundraising capacity..." from competition by survivor groups. Not surprisingly, the authoritative U.S. charity watchdog, *the Chronicle of Philanthropy*, warned against the transfer of money from the public purse to private hands. *The ACS is more interested in accumulating wealth than saving lives.*

These conflicts of interest extended to the personal. The legislative committee cochair, DeVita, was board chairman of CancerSource.com, a website promoting the ACS *Consumers' Guide to Cancer Drugs*. As disturbing, DeVita and Dr. John Mendelsohn, director of the NCI's MD Anderson Comprehensive Cancer Center, were consultants and board members of the publicly traded cancer drug company, ImClone Systems, Inc. Mendelsohn was also a board member of Enron, besides serving on its Audit Committee; Enron was a generous and long-term supporter of the M.D. Anderson. In May 2001 television and radio interviews, DeVita expressed enthusiasm on cancer drugs that targeted "EGF" receptors. However, he failed to disclose his annual $100,000 consulting fees from ImClone which was then actively seeking FDA approval of its targeted cancer drug Erbitux. DeVita also insisted, contrary to NCI's own data, that the overall incidence of cancer had been decreasing at a steep rate every year since 1990. In May 2002, Dr. Samuel Waksal resigned as president and CEO of ImClone. One month later, he was arrested on charges of criminal conspiracy, securities fraud and perjury, and civil damages for insider trading and was subsequently indicted on charges of insider trading, bank fraud, forging a signature and obstructing a federal investigation.

In the September/October 2002 issue of the *Cancer Journal*, an article by its coeditor DeVita, "A Perspective on the War on Cancer" was prefaced by the following disclaimer: "No benefits in any form have been or will be received from a commercial party related directly or indirectly to the subject of this article." However, as pointed out in a November 15, 2002, letter (by the author) to the *Journal*'s other coeditors, Drs. Samuel Hellman and Steven Rosenberg, this disclaimer was inconsistent with DeVita's conflicts of interest relating to the CancerSource.com website and his ImClone consulting fees. The editors of the *Journal* responded that it "takes matters of conflict of interest and disclosure very seriously" but, nevertheless, declined to publish the letter.

ACS has interlocking interests with the pharmaceutical, cancer drug, mammography film and machine, and biotechnology industries. This is reflected by generous ACS allocations for research on highly profitable patented cancer drugs and aggressive promotion of premenopausal mammography. In striking contrast, less than 0.1% of revenues in 1998 were allocated to environmental, occupational, and other avoidable causes of cancer. More seriously, ACS policies on primary cancer prevention extend from a decades-long track record of indifference, or even hostility, compounded by proindustry bias, even to the tobacco industry. Shandwick International, representing RJ Reynolds, and Edelman Worldwide, representing Brown & Williamson Tobacco Company, have been major PR firms for the ACS; Shandwick assisted the NDC in drafting the new National Cancer Act while Edelman conducted the ACS voter-education campaign for the 2000 presidential elections. ACS promptly discontinued these relations, protesting "front end due diligence," once the damaging information became public.

The highly politicized and nontransparent agenda of the ACS is troubling. This is further exemplified by expenditures on lobbying, including donations to Democratic and Republican Governors' associations: "We wanted to look like players and be players," an ACS representative admitted. Tax experts have warned that these contributions may be illegal as charities are not allowed to make political donations. Marcus Owen, director of the IRS Exempt Organization Division, also warned, "The bottom line is campaign contributions will jeopardize a charity's exempt status."

It should be emphasized that the ACS has long exercised dominant influence over NCI policy and remains "the tail that wags the NCI dog." This influence was consolidated by the February 2002 appointment of Dr. Andrew von Eschenbach as NCI director; prior to his appointment, Eschenbach was vice president of the MD Anderson Cancer Center and president-elect of the ACS. Furthermore, as a condition of his appointment, Eschenbach obtained agreement that he continue as NDC's leader. Thus, irrespective of the Feinstein initiative, to all intents and purposes, the National Cancer Program has since become privatized.

HIDDEN CONFLICTS
OF INTEREST

Public Relations

- 1998-2000: PR for the ACS was handled by Shandwick International, whose major clients included RJ Reynolds Tobacco Holdings.
- 2000-2002: PR for the ACS was handled by Edelman Public Relations, whose major clients included Brown & Williamson Tobacco Company, the Altria Group, the parent company of Philip Morris, Kraft, and fast-food and soft drink beverage companies.

Industry Funding

ACS has received contributions in excess of $100,000 from a wide range of "Excalibur donors." Some of these companies were responsible for environmental pollution with carcinogens while others manufactured and sold products containing toxic and carcinogenic ingredients. These include as follows:

- Petrochemical companies (DuPont, BP, and Pennzoil)
- Industrial waste companies (BFI Waste Systems)
- Big Pharma (AstraZeneca, Bristol-Myers Squibb, GlaxoSmithKline, Merck & Company, and Novartis)
- Auto companies (Nissan and General Motors)
- Cosmetic companies (Christian Dior, Avon, Revlon, and Elizabeth Arden)

- Junk food companies (Wendy's International, McDonalds's, Unilever/Best Foods, and Coca-Cola)
- Biotech companies (Amgen and Genentech)

Nevertheless, as reported in the December 8, 2009, *New York Times*, the ACS claims that it "holds itself to the highest standards of transparency and public accountability."

Reckless, If Not Criminal, Track Record on Cancer Prevention*

1971 When studies unequivocally proved that diethylstilbestrol (DES) caused vaginal cancers in teenage daughters of women administered the drug during pregnancy, the ACS refused an invitation to testify at Congressional hearings to require the U.S. Food and Drug Administration (FDA) to ban its use as an animal feed additive. It gave no reason for its refusal. Not surprisingly, U.S. meat is banned by other nations worldwide.

1977 The ACS opposed regulations proposed for hair-coloring products that contained dyes known to cause breast and liver cancer in rodents. In so doing, the ACS ignored virtually every tenet of responsible public health as these chemicals were clear-cut liver and breast carcinogens.

The ACS also called for a congressional moratorium on the FDA's proposed ban on saccharin and even advocated its use by nursing mothers and babies in moderation despite clear-cut evidence of its carcinogenicity in

---

* Based in part on THE STOP CANCER BEFORE IT STARTS CAMPAIGN: How to Win the Losing War against Cancer (Cancer Prevention Coalition Report, 2003). This report was sponsored by eight leading cancer prevention experts, endorsed by over a hundred activists and citizen groups, and is based in part on a prior publication in the International Journal of Health Services (see appendix A).

rodents. This reflects the consistent rejection by the ACS of the importance of animal evidence as predictive of human cancer risk.

1978   Tony Mazzocchi, then senior representative of the Oil, Chemical, and Atomic Workers International Union, stated at a Washington, D.C., roundtable between public interest groups and high-ranking ACS officials: "Occupational safety standards have received no support from the ACS." Congressman Paul Rogers also censured the ACS for doing "too little, too late" in failing to support the Clean Air Act.

1982   The ACS adopted a highly restrictive cancer policy that insisted on unequivocal human evidence of carcinogenicity before taking any position on public health hazards. Accordingly, the ACS still trivializes or rejects evidence of carcinogenicity in experimental animals and has actively campaigned against laws (the 1958 Delaney Law, for instance) that ban deliberate addition to food of any amount of any additive shown to cause cancer in either animals or humans. The ACS still persists in an anti-Delaney policy despite the overwhelming support for this law by the independent scientific community.

1983   The ACS refused to join a coalition of the March of Dimes, American Heart Association, and the American Lung Association to support the Clear Air Act.

1984   The ACS created the October National Breast Cancer Awareness Month, funded and promoted by Zeneca, an offshoot of the UK Imperial Chemical Industry, a major manufacturer of petrochemical products. The ACS leads women to believe that mammography is their best hope against breast cancer. A recent ACS advertisement promised that "early detection results in a cure nearly 100% of the time." Responding to questions from a journalist, an ACS communications director admitted, "The ad is based on a study. When you make an advertisement, you just say what you can to get women in the door. You exaggerate a point. Mammography today is a lucrative [and] highly competitive business." Even more seriously, the awareness month publications and advertisements studiously avoid any reference to the wealth of information on avoidable causes and prevention of breast cancer.

1989   Launched in 1989 by the Cosmetic, Toiletry, and Fragrance Association (CTFA) and the National Cosmetology Association, the Look Good . . . Feel Better Program was "dedicated to teaching women cancer patients beauty techniques to help restore their appearance and self-image during cancer treatment."

Just what could be more noble? Or so it might just seem. The October 2005 Look Good Program was supported by twenty-two CTFA-member cosmetic companies, including multibillion-dollar household name global giants. Each year, member companies "donate over one million individual cosmetic and personal care products, valued at $10 million, and raise more than $2 million." The program was administered nationwide by the ACS, "which managed volunteer training, and served as the primary source of information to the public."

There is no doubt that the products donated by the cosmetic companies—such as eye and cheek colors, lipsticks, moisture lotions, pressed powders, and other makeup—are restorative. However, there is also no doubt that the ACS and the companies involved were oblivious to or strangely silent on the dangers of the Look Good products, whose ingredients were readily absorbed through the skin.

A review of twelve Look Good products, marketed by six companies, revealed that ten contained toxic ingredients. These pose risks of cancer and also hormonal (endocrine disruptive) effects.

Evidence for the cancer risks is based on standard tests in rodents and on human (epidemiological) studies. Evidence for the hormonal risks is based on test-tube tests with breast cancer cells or by stimulating premature sexual development in infant rodents. Unbelievably, the ACS explicitly warns women undergoing cancer chemotherapy—"Don't use hormonal creams."

Take for example Estee Lauder's Light Source Transforming Moisture Lotion, Chanel's Sheer Lipstick, and Merle Norman Eye Color. These products contain ingredients that are carcinogenic, contaminated with carcinogens, or precursors of carcinogens. The products also contain hormonal ingredients, known as parabens, one of which has been identified in breast cancer tissue and incriminated as a probable cause of breast cancer.

The ACS's silence with regard to the risks of the Look Good products extends more widely to cosmetics and personal care products used by women, personal care products used by men, and baby lotions and shampoos. This silence is also consistent with the imbalanced objectives of the ACS highly publicized annual Breast Cancer Awareness Month. While dedicated to the early detection of breast cancer, this event is silent on a wide range of its avoidable causes, besides the escalating incidence of postmenopausal breast cancer, by nearly 40% over the last three decades.

Of likely relevance to the ACS silence is its interlocking interests with the cosmetic, besides other industries. The major Look Good companies were among some 350 ACS "Excalibur donors," each donating a minimum of $10,000 annually. Other donors include petrochemical, power plant, and hazardous waste industries, whose environmental pollutants have been incriminated as causes of breast, besides other, cancers.

The ACS's silence was also recklessly shared by the National Cancer Institute (NCI), which is required by the 1971 National Cancer Act to provide the public with information on avoidable causes of cancer. However, despite approximately $50 billion of taxpayers funding since 1971, the NCI has joined with the ACS in denying the public's right to know of avoidable causes of cancer from industrial chemicals, radiation, and common prescription drugs. Both the NCI and ACS are locked at the hip in policies fixated on damage control-screening, diagnosis, treatment and treatment-related research, with indifference to cancer prevention due to avoidable exposures to chemical carcinogens in cosmetics, other consumer products, air and water.

Equally asleep at the wheel remained the Food and Drug Administration despite its regulatory authority. The 1938 Federal Food, Drug, and Cosmetic Act explicitly requires that "the label of cosmetic products shall bear a warning statement . . . to prevent a health hazard that may be associated with a product."

1992 The ACS issued a joint statement with the Chlorine Institute in support of the continued global use of organochlorine pesticides despite clear evidence that some were known to cause breast cancer. In this statement, ACS vice president Clark Heath, MD, dismissed evidence of any risk as "preliminary and mostly based on weak and indirect association." Heath then went on to explain away the blame for increasing breast cancer rates as due to better detection: "Speculation that such exposures account for observed geographic differences in breast cancer occurrence should be received with caution; more likely, much of the recent rise in incidence in the United States . . . reflects increased utilization of mammography over the past decade."

In conjunction with the NCI, the ACS aggressively launched a "chemoprevention" program aimed at recruiting 16,000 healthy women at supposedly "high risk" of breast cancer into a five-year clinical trial with a highly profitable drug called Tamoxifen. This drug is manufactured by one of the world's most powerful cancer drug industries, Zeneca, an offshoot of the Imperial Chemical Industries. The women were told that the drug was essentially harmless and that it could reduce their risk of breast cancer. What the women were not told was that Tamoxifen had already been shown to be a highly potent liver carcinogen in rodent tests and was also well-known to induce uterine cancer in women.

1993 Just before PBS *Frontline* aired the special titled, "In Our Children's Food," the ACS came out in support of the pesticide industry. In a damage-control memorandum sent to some forty-eight regional divisions and their three thousand local offices, the ACS trivialized pesticides as a cause of childhood cancer. The ACS also reassured the public that carcinogenic pesticide residues in food are safe, even for babies. When the media and concerned citizens called local ACS chapters, they received reassurances crafted by Porter Novelli, a powerful PR firm for the agribusiness industry, and then rehashed and sent to another client, the ACS:

> The primary health hazards of pesticides are from direct contact with the chemicals at potentially high doses, for example, farm workers who apply the chemicals and work in the fields after the pesticides have been applied, and people living near aerially sprayed fields . . . . The American Cancer Society believes that the benefits of a balanced diet rich in fruits and vegetables far outweigh the largely theoretical risks posed by occasional, very low pesticide residue levels in foods.

In support of this ACS agribusiness initiative, these reassurances were then rehashed for a third time by the right-wing group, Accuracy in Media (AIM), which published quotes from the ACS memorandum in an article with the banner headline: "Junk Science on PBS," with an opening, "Can we afford the Public Broadcasting Services?"

Based on these and other, long-standing concerns, the *Chronicle of Philanthropy*, the nation's leading charity watchdog, published a statement that "the ACS is more interested in accumulating wealth than saving lives."

1994 The ACS published a study designed to reassure women on the safety of dark permanent hair dyes and trivialize risks of fatal and nonfatal cancers as documented in over six prior reports. However, the ACS study was based on a group of some 1,100 women with an initial age of fifty-six who were followed for seven years only. The ACS concluded that "women using permanent hair dyes are not generally at increased risk of fatal cancer." However, risks of cancer in women over sixty-three are up to twenty times higher for non-Hodgkin's lymphoma and multiple myeloma, thirty-four times for bladder cancer, and eight times for breast cancer. As designed, the ACS study would have missed the great majority of these cancers and excluded dark hair dyes as important risks of avoidable cancers.

The ACS abysmal track record on prevention has been and remains the subject of periodic protests by leading independent scientists and public interest groups. A well-publicized example was a New York City, January 23, 1994, press conference, sponsored by the author and the Center for Science in the Public Interest. Their press release stated, "A group of 24 scientists charged that the ACS was doing little to protect the public from cancer-causing chemicals in the environment and workplace. The scientists urged ACS to revamp its policies and to emphasize prevention in its lobbying and educational campaigns." The scientists—including—Harvard University Nobel laureates Matthew Meselson and George Wald; former Occupational Safety and Health director Eula Bingham; Samuel Epstein, author of the *Politics of Cancer*; and Anthony Robbins, past president of the American Public Health Association—criticized the ACS for insisting on unequivocal human evidence that an exposure or chemical is carcinogenic before it would recommend its regulation.

This public criticism by a broad representation of highly credible scientists reflected the well-established conviction that a substantial proportion of cancer deaths are caused by exposure to chemical carcinogens in the air, water, food supply, and workplace, all of which could be prevented by legislative and regulatory action. Calling the ACS guidelines an "unrealistically high-action threshold," a letter from the January 1994 scientists to ACS executive vice president Lane Adams stated that "we would like to express our hope that ACS will take strong public positions and become a more active force to protect the public and the work force from exposure to carcinogens."

However, ACS's policies remain retrogressive and contrary to authoritative and scientific tenets established by international and national scientific committees and also in conflict with long-established policies of federal regulatory agencies. Speakers at the 1994 press conference also warned that unless the ACS became more supportive of cancer prevention, it would face the risk of an economic boycott. Reacting promptly, the ACS issued a statement claiming that cancer prevention would then become a major priority. However, ACS policies have remained unchanged.

1996   The ACS, together with a diverse group of patient and physician organizations, filed a citizen's petition to pressure the FDA to ease restrictions on access to silicone gel breast implants. What the ACS did not disclose was that the gel in these implants had clearly been shown to induce cancer in several rodent studies and also that these implants were contaminated with other potent carcinogens such as ethylene oxide and crystalline silica.

1998   In *Cancer Facts & Figures—1998*, the annual ACS publication designed to provide the public and medical profession with basic facts on cancer, there is little or no mention of prevention. Examples include dusting the genital area with talc as a known cause of ovarian cancer; no mention of parental exposure to occupational carcinogens as a major cause of childhood cancer; prolonged use of oral contraceptives and hormone replacement therapy as major causes of breast cancer. For breast cancer, ACS stated, "Since women may not be able to alter their personal risk factors, the best opportunity for reducing mortality is through early detection." In other words, breast cancer is not preventable despite clear evidence that its incidence had escalated over recent decades and despite an overwhelming literature on its avoidable causes. In the section on "Nutrition and Diet," no mention is made of the heavy contamination of animal and dairy fats and produce with a wide range of carcinogenic pesticide residues and on the need to switch to safer organic foods.

The ACS allocated $330,000, under 0.1% of its $678 million revenues, to research on Environmental Carcinogenesis while claiming allocations of $2.6 million, 0.4% of its revenues. Furthermore, in its annual publication, *Cancer Facts & Figures*—designed to provide the public and medical profession with basic facts on cancer other than information on incidence, mortality, and treatment—there was little or no mention of primary prevention. For breast cancer, ACS stated, "Since women may not be able to alter their personal risk factors, the best opportunity for reducing mortality is through early detection."

1999   The ACS denied any risks of cancer from drinking genetically-engineered (rBGH) milk. Its position has remained unchanged despite strong scientific evidence relating rBGH milk to major risks of breast, prostate, and colon cancers as detailed in my 2006 *What's in Your Milk?* book (Trafford Publishing, 2006).

CANCER	AUTHOR	EXCESS RISKS
BREAST	Bruning et al., 1995	7.3
	Hankinson et al., 1998	7.3
	Del Giudice et al., 1998	2.1
PROSTATE	Signorello et al., 1999	5.1
	Chan et al., 1998	4.3
	Mantzoros et al., 1997	1.9
	Wolk et al., 1995	1.4
COLON	Pollak et al., 1999	5.0
	Manousos et al., 1999	2.7
	Ma et al., 1999	2.5
	Giovanucci et al., 1999	2.2

Evidence for these risks is also summarized in my May 11, 2007, and January 12, 2010, Citizen Petitions to the Food and Drug Administration. These requested the FDA commissioner "to label milk and other dairy products produced with the use of Posilac with a cancer risk warning." Both petitions were endorsed by leading national experts and supported by over sixty scientific references. However, the FDA has still remained recklessly unresponsive.

2000 The January *Cancer Letter*, commented on the behind-the-scenes ACS creation of a legislative committee to gain major control of national cancer policy. Dr. John Durant, former executive president of the American Society of Clinical Oncologists, charged, "It has always seemed to me that was an issue of control by the ACS over the cancer agenda. They are protecting their own fundraising capacity . . ." from competition by survivor groups.

Also, the *Cancer Letter* revealed that ACS public relations had close ties to the tobacco industry. Shandwick International, representing RJ Reynolds Tobacco Holdings, and subsequently by Edelman Public Relations, representing Brown & Williamson Tobacco Company, had been major public relations firms for the ACS in its attempts to rewrite the 1971 National Cancer Act, and in conducting voter education programs in the past presidential campaign.

2002 In the *ACS Cancer Facts and Figures 2002*, the Community Cancer Control Section includes a Look Good . . . Feel Better program to teach women cancer patients beauty techniques to help restore their appearance and self-image during chemotherapy and radiation treatment. This program was partnered by the National Cosmetology Association and the Cosmetic, Toiletry, and Fragrance Association Foundation, which failed to disclose the wide range of carcinogenic ingredients in toiletries and cosmetics. These trade organizations have also failed to disclose evidence of excess risks of breast and other cancers following long-term use of black or dark brown permanent and semi-permanent hair dyes. *The ACS also failed to inform women of these avoidable risks.*

The Environmental Cancer Risk Section of the *ACS Facts and Figures Report* also reassured that carcinogenic exposures from dietary pesticides, "toxic wastes in dump sites," ionizing radiation from "closely controlled" nuclear power plants and nonionizing radiation, are all "at such low levels that risks are negligible."

2005 The ACS indifference to cancer prevention other than smoking remained unchanged despite the escalating incidence of cancer and its $1 billion budget. Some of the more startling realities in the failure to prevent cancers are illustrated by their soaring increases from 1975 to 2005 based on NCI epidemiological data.

2007   The ACS's indifference to cancer prevention has remained unchanged despite evidence on the escalating incidence of a wide range of cancers for over three decades.

Incidence Rates for Major Cancers, 1975-2007

CANCERS	% Increase
Childhood (ages 0-19)	30
Non-Hodgkin's Lymphoma	82
Acute Lymphocytic Leukemia:	67
Female Breast: Postmenopausal	23
Testes	60
Thyroid	145
Melanoma	163
Kidney and Renal Pelvis	107
Lung	
Overall	13
Male	-22
Female	110
All Sites	15

Some of the more startling realities in the failure of the ACS to recognize and warn of the escalating incidence of a wide range of avoidable cancers, as documented in the National Toxicology Program (NTP) and International Agency for Research on Cancer (IARC) reports, is illustrated by their soaring incidence from 1975. These include as follows:

• Childhood cancer. This increased by 30% due to ionizing radiation; domestic pesticides; nitrite preservatives in meats, particularly hot dogs; and parental exposures to occupational carcinogens.

- Non-Hodgkin's lymphoma. This increased by 82% due mostly to phenoxy herbicides and phenylenediamine hair dyes.
- Postmenopausal breast cancer. This increased by 23% due to a wide range of known causes. These include birth control pills, estrogen replacement therapy, toxic hormonal ingredients in cosmetics and personal care products, diagnostic radiation, and routine premenopausal mammography, with a cumulative breast dose exposure of up to about five rads over ten years.
- Testes cancer. This increased by 60% due to pesticides, hormonal ingredients in cosmetics and personal care products, and estrogen residues in meat.
- Malignant melanoma in adults. This increased by 163% due to the use of sunscreens in childhood that fail to block long wave ultraviolet light.

2009 The ACS 2009 budget was about $1 billion, of which 17% was allotted to prevention, predominantly smoking cessation, and 28% to support services and salaries. The top three executive salaries listed ranged from $670,000 to $1.2 million.

In a 2009 publication by Dr. Elizabeth Fontham titled "American Cancer Society Perspectives on Environmental Factors and Cancer," she claimed that "cancer prevention is central to the ACS and are primarily focused on modifiable risk factors that have been demonstrated to have the largest impact on cancer risk in the general population, with particular emphasis on tobacco, and well-proven policy and program interventions. The ACS addresses nutrition, physical inactivity and obesity, alcohol consumption, excessive sun exposure, prevention of certain chronic infections, and selected other environmental factors through a variety of venues." Dr. Fontham also reiterated long-standing ACS claims that "the estimated percentage of cancers related to occupational and environmental carcinogens is small compared to the cancer burden from tobacco smoking (30%) and the combination of nutrition, physical activity, and obesity (35%)."

2010 On May 6, 2010, the President's Cancer Panel released an approximately two hundred-page report, "REDUCING ENVIRONMENTAL CANCER: What We Can Do Now."

Meticulously documented and with comprehensive scientific references, the Cancer Panel report warned, "Though overall cancer incidence and mortality have continued to decline in recent years, the disease continues to devastate the lives of far too many Americans. In 2009 alone, approximately 1.5 million American men, women, and children were diagnosed with cancer, and 562,000 died from the disease. With the growing body of evidence linking environmental exposures to cancer, the public is becoming increasingly aware of the unacceptable burden of cancer resulting from environmental and occupational exposures that could have been prevented through appropriate national action. The Administration's commitment to the cancer community and recent focus on critically needed reform of the Toxic Substances Control Act is praiseworthy. However, our Nation still has much work ahead to identify the many existing but unrecognized environmental carcinogens and eliminate those that are known from our workplaces, schools, and homes."

"The [President's] Panel was particularly concerned to find that the true burden of environmentally induced cancer has been grossly underestimated. With nearly 80,000 chemicals on the market in the United States, many of which are used by millions of Americans in their daily lives and are un—or understudied and largely unregulated, exposure to potential environmental carcinogens is widespread." The panel concluded that cancer caused by environmental exposure has been "grossly underestimated." The panel also listed a wide range of cancers, such as breast, kidney, leukemia, liver, and non-Hodgkin's lymphoma for which well-documented causes are detailed.

Appendix F of the panel is a masterly and comprehensive summary of known strong and suspected carcinogens, their sources/uses, and their strong or suspected links to specified cancers. This appendix is an update of a publication by Dr. Richard Clapp, an internationally recognized expert on avoidable causes of cancer, in the prestigious 2008 *Reviews of Environmental Health*.

The President's Report was promptly endorsed by a wide range of leading scientific and public policy experts. The report also lent strong support to Senator Frank Lautenberg's Safe Chemicals Act of 2010 intended to ensure the safety of all chemicals used in commerce.

In July 2010, just two months following its rejection of the President's Report, the ACS released a publication by Dr. Elizabeth Ward, ACS vice president of Epidemiology and Surveillance Research, titled "Research Recommendations for Selected High-Priority IARC (International Agency for Research on Cancer) Carcinogens." This focused on "twenty agents—prioritized for review in occupational populations." Trying to play both sides, Dr. Ward conceded that "there is more of a hint that in most cases (these carcinogens) might be involved with cancer." Nevertheless, she dismissively claimed that "the studies that could make a definitive link are missing and need more study." She also claimed that while there is significant concern about substances or exposures in the environment that may cause cancer, there are some agents and exposure circumstances where evidence of carcinogenicity is substantial, but not yet conclusive.

Dr. Ward's qualified publication hardly is surprising. Only two months previously, the ACS had explicitly dismissed scientific evidence on the carcinogens previously identified in appendix F of the President's Cancer Panel Report. However, this evidence had been fully documented in 2004 by the Department of Health and Human Services National Toxicology Program (NTP), besides confirmed by other U.S. federal agencies, besides the International Agency for Research on Cancer (IARC).

The President's Cancer Panel Report was also promptly criticized by Dr. Michael Thun, ACS vice president emeritus, in his 2010 publication, "The Global Burden of Cancer: Priorities for Prevention." "Unfortunately, the perspective of the report is unbalanced by its implication that pollution is the major cause of cancer, and by its dismissal of cancer prevention efforts aimed at the major known causes of cancer (tobacco, obesity, alcohol, infections, hormones, sunlight) as focused narrowly." These exclusionary and self-interested claims had also been expressed by Dr. Elizabeth Fontham, ACS vice president in epidemiology research, in her 2009 publication, "American Cancer Society Perspectives on Environmental Factors and Cancer."

The ACS further complained that it would be unfortunate if people came away with the message that the chemicals in the environment are the most important cause of cancer at the expense of those lifestyle factors—like tobacco, physical activity, nutrition, and obesity—that have, by far, the most potential in reducing cancer deaths.

"Elements of this report are entirely consistent with the recently published 'American Cancer Society Perspective on Environmental Factors and Cancer' which, like the current report, identifies several areas of particular concern."

These concerns "include the accumulation of certain chemicals in humans and in the food chain, especially those that mimic naturally occurring hormones or other processes in the body; the potentially greater susceptibility of children and other subgroups; the large number of industrial chemicals that have not been adequately tested for toxicity and carcinogenicity; potential cancer risks from widely used medical imaging procedures that involve ionizing radiation; potential biological effects of chemicals at low doses; and the potential effects of combinations of exposures.

"In fact, the precise proportion of cancers related to environmental exposure has been debated for nearly 30 years. And while there is no doubt exposure to chemicals has some bearing on cancer risk, the level of risk is certainly far below other identified cancer risks, like tobacco, nutrition, physical activity, and obesity.

"There is no doubt that environmental pollution is critically important to the health of humans and the planet. However, it would be unfortunate if the effects of this report were to trivialize the importance of other modifiable risk factors that offer the greatest opportunity in preventing cancer.

"The [President's Cancer Panel] report is most provocative when it restates hypotheses as if they were established fact. For example, its conclusion that the true burden of environmentally (i.e. pollution) induced cancer has been grossly underestimated does not represent scientific consensus. Rather, it reflects one side of a scientific debate that has continued for almost 30 years."

Of inescapable and incriminatory concern, the ACS admission on the predominant role on these avoidable causes of cancer is decades overdue. The ACS cannot escape unarguable, if not criminal, responsibility for the countless avoidable nonsmoking-related cancers and deaths.

From its inception in 1922 until now, the public has been and continues to be misled by the ACS and, most recently, by Drs. Thun and Ward, with their exclusionary emphasis on personal responsibility and faulty lifestyle as the predominant cause of cancer. However, this reckless misrepresentation contrasts bizarrely with their two scientific publications in 2009 and one in June this year, incriminating a wide range of avoidable environmental causes of cancer and priorities for its prevention. However, the public still remains uninformed of these belated and damaging admissions responsible for countless cancers and deaths over the last nine decades.

Criticism by the Society of Toxicology

The August 6, 2010, *Cancer Letter* published a letter from the Society of Toxicology, which traditionally has faithfully endorsed ACS policies, criticizing the May 6 President's Cancer Panel Report.

"The Society of Toxicology applauds this effort to raise awareness of environmental causes of cancer, and supports the need to understand the role that environmental factors play in this disease.

"The Panel's report has been received with mixed reviews from some medical and scientific experts as well as several organizations and advocacy groups. For example, while experts generally believe that the increasing number of known or suspected environmental carcinogens warrants further study and action to reduce or eliminate these exposures, some are concerned that the report overstates the risk of environmentally-induced cancer and gives too little attention to the major known causes of cancer, including tobacco, obesity, sunlight, and alcohol.

"A second criticism is that the report recommends a precautionary approach. The SOT is firmly committed to disease prevention as noted by one of the Society's strategic objectives, "Increase the impact of toxicology on human health and disease prevention." However, THE SOT claims that at the heart of toxicological research is the premise that "the dose makes the poison." So we believe that current regulatory decisions should be based on well-informed safety assessments that emphasize appropriate dose-response data." In this connection, the SOT is on record as fighting against the 1958 Delaney Amendment to the 1938 Federal Food Drug and Cosmetic Act. This requires an automatic ban on food additives causing cancer in experimental animals or men. In a similar class, the American Conference of Governmental Industrial Hygienists has generated so-called safe exposure levels or "threshold limit values," exposure levels for carcinogens.

ACS Cancer Facts and Figures 2010 Annual Report

Can Cancer Be Prevented?

"All cancers caused by cigarette smoking and heavy use of alcohol could be prevented completely. The American Cancer Society estimates that in 2010, 171,000 cancer deaths are expected to be caused by tobacco use. Scientific evidence suggests that about one-third of the 569,490 cancer deaths expected to occur in 2010 will be related to overweight or obesity, physical inactivity, and poor nutrition and thus could also be prevented. Certain cancers are related to infectious agents, such as hepatitis B virus (HBV), human papilloma virus (HPV), human immunodeficiency virus (HIV), Helicobacter pylori (H. pylori), and others, and could be prevented through behavioral changes, vaccines, or antibiotics. In addition, many of the more than 1 million skin cancers that are expected to be diagnosed in 2010 could be prevented by protection from the sun's rays and avoiding indoor tanning.

"Regular screening examinations by a health care professional can result in the detection and removal of precancerous growths, as well as the diagnosis of cancers at an early stage, when they are most treatable. Cancers that can be prevented by removal of precancerous tissue include cancers of the cervix, colon, and rectum. Cancers that can be diagnosed early through screening include cancers of the breast, colon, rectum, cervix, prostate, oral cavity, and skin. For cancers of breast, colon, rectum, and cervix, early detection has been proven to reduce mortality. A heightened awareness of breast changes or skin changes may also result in detection of these tumors at earlier stages. Cancers that can be prevented or detected earlier by screening account for at least half of all new cancer cases."

Strikingly, this 2010 report, like its five annual predecessors, avoids any reference to eleven carcinogens identified in the 2004 National Toxicology Program (NTP) Report, besides nine of the same also identified in the 2010 President's Cancer Panel (PCP) Report. More substantively, this report raises serious concerns as to whether the ACS remains fixated on its decades old insistence on "blame the victim" responsibility for avoidable causes of cancer.

Carcinogens Listed in the 2010 American Cancer Society (ACS) Report as "Needing More Study," But Previously Identified as Carcinogens and by the 2010 President's Cancer Panel (PCP) Report and by the 2004 National Toxicology Program (NTP) *11th Report On Carcinogens*

Carcinogens	NTP (2004)*	PCP (2010)**
Lead and Lead compounds	+	+
Diesel exhaust	+	++
Styrene-7,8-oxide and styrene	+	+
Propylene oxide	+	
Formaldehyde	+	++
Acetaldehyde	+	
Methylene chloride	+	+
Trichloroethylene	+	++
Tetrachloroethylene	+	+
Chloroform	+	++
Polychlorinated biphenyls	+	++

NTP RATING
Reasonably anticipated   +

**PCP RATING*
Strong   + +
Suspected   +

2011   On February 18, the ACS stated that it has "no formal position regarding rBGH [in milk]" and that "the evidence for potential harm to humans is inconclusive." The ACS also claimed that "while there may be a link between IGF-1 levels in milk and cancer, the exact nature of this link remains unclear." This claim is contrary to the unequivocal evidence of increased risks of breast, colon, and prostate cancers (see 1999 track record).

INTERNATIONAL RELAY
FOR LIFE

Since 1996, the ACS has collaborated with cancer organizations in about ninety countries outside the United States to license and support its Relay for Life programs (http://www.relayforlife.org/relay). The international relay "enables cancer leagues around the globe to increase their visibility and income—while building survivorship, volunteerism, and advocacy efforts in their communities."

As the ACS states, its "International Relay for Life is a training and technical assistance program for cancer organizations worldwide." Team members take turns to walk or run around a track for twelve to twenty-four hours. "Through the Relay, these organizations bring together passionate volunteers, promote their mission-based activities, and mobilize communities to take action in the international movement to end cancer" by stopping smoking and developing health lifestyles. "No matter where they take place in the world, Relay events are intended to give people a chance to celebrate the lives of cancer survivors, remember loved ones lost, and fight back against a disease that has taken too much."

In each of over ninety relay nations, "the funds support local organizations' cancer control programs, services, and research. These organizations also contribute part of their funds to the Global Cancer Fund, which supports ACS cancer control programs in developing countries that would not otherwise be possible."

In the 2010 Relay for Life, ninety nations worldwide celebrated 14 years of "helping save lives from cancer." However, the future of the Relays now depends on whether the ACS belatedly becomes more interested in saving lives than accumulating wealth.

ACS Press Releases and Huffington Post Blogs

October 14, 1994	Breast Cancer Unawareness Month
October 18, 1995	National Mammography Day
April 1, 1998	Cancer Report Card Gets a Failing Grade
August 25, 1998	The Cancer Drug Industry "March" Seriously Misleads the Nation
October 26, 1999	American Cancer Society Indicted for Losing the Winnable War against Cancer
May 30, 2000	American Cancer Society: Long on Promise, Short on Delivery
June 12, 2001	The American Cancer Society Is Threatening the National Cancer Program
May 9, 2002	Escalating Incidence of Childhood Cancer Is Ignored by the National Cancer Institute and American Cancer Society
February 25, 2003	National Cancer Institute Leadership Is out of Touch with Reality
May 23, 2003	The American Cancer Society Misleads the Public in the May 26 Discovery Health Channel Program
February 23, 2004	Spinning the Losing Cancer War
February 28, 2005	Time to Protect Babies from Dangerous Products
October 28, 2005	The Look Good . . . Feel Better Program. But at What Risk?
October 16, 2007	Breast Cancer Awareness Month Misleads Women
July 22, 2009	Safe Breast Self Exam by Young Women Vs. Dangers of Mammography

October 14, 1994

BREAST CANCER UNAWARENESS MONTH

Commenting on the anniversary of National Breast Cancer Awareness month (NBCAM), Dr. Samuel Epstein, Chairman of the Cancer Prevention Coalition (CPC) stated, "A decade-old multi-million dollar deal between National Breast Cancer Awareness Month sponsors and Imperial Chemical Industries (ICI) has produced reckless misinformation on breast cancer." Dr. Epstein, a leading international authority on cancer causing effects of environmental pollutants, will be speaking on breast cancer prevention at a conference, "Women, Health, & the Environment" in Albuquerque, New Mexico on October 14-15. It is sponsored by CPC, in conjunction with Greenpeace and Women's Environmental and Development Organization (WEDO).

Zeneca Pharmaceutical, a U.S. subsidiary and recent spinoff of ICI, has been the sole founder of National Breast Cancer Awareness Month since 1984. ICI is one of the largest manufacturers of petrochemical and chlorinated organic products, such as acetochlor and vinyl chloride, and the sole manufacturer of Tamoxifen, the world's top-selling cancer drug used for breast cancer. Financial sponsorship by Zeneca/ICI gives them editorial control over every leaflet, poster, publication, and commercial produced by NBCAM. NBCAM is promoted by the cancer establishment, the National Cancer Institute (NCI) and the American Cancer Society (ACS) with their corporate sponsors.

ICI has supported the NCI/ACS blame-the-victim theory of the causes of breast and other cancers. This theory attributes escalating cancer rates to heredity and faulty lifestyle, rather than avoidable exposures to industrial carcinogens contaminating air, water, food, consumer products, and the workplace.

Dr. Epstein will summarize the evidence on avoidable environmental and other causes of breast cancer ignored in NBCAM promotional materials:

- Since the 1950's scientific evidence has incriminated chlorinated organic pesticides as breast cancer risk factors because of their carcinogenicity, estrogenic effects, and accumulation in body fat, particularly the breast.
- The unregulated use of growth promoting hormonal cattle feed additives has resulted in near universal contamination of meat products. This results in life-long exposure to carcinogenic estrogens, and poses a major avoidable risk of breast cancer.

- Where you work increases your breast cancer risks. Excess breast cancers were found in the 1970's in women working with vinyl chloride. There is similar evidence among petrochemical and electrical workers. In spite of more women working in such industries, NCI recently admitted that it has still not investigated these risks among working women.

- Where you live increases risks of breast cancer. Based on a review of 21 New Jersey counties, and more recently 339 nationwide counties, statistically significant associations were found between excess breast cancer mortality and residence in counties where hazardous waste sites are located.

- Living near a nuclear facility increases your chances of dying from breast cancer. Based on a nationwide survey of 268 counties within 50 miles of 51 military and civilian nuclear reactors, CPC member Dr. Jay Gould, showed that breast cancer mortality in these "nuclear counties" has increased at 10 times the national rate from 1950 to 1989. Counties near military reactors, such as Hanford, Oak Ridge and Savannah River, have registered the greatest increases, ranging from 27 to 200%. Dr. Gould charged NCI with "misrepresentation of such findings."

- Premenopausal mammography increases your risk of breast cancer. Increases in breast cancer mortality have been consistently reported following repeated mammograms in younger women in six randomized controlled clinical trials over the last decade. Based on this evidence, NCI has recently withdrawn recommendations for pre-menopausal mammography. ACS, with financial support from Dupont and General Electric (both heavily invested in mammography equipment), and self-interested radiologists are still promoting this dangerous practice.

- Participation in the 1972 NCI/ACS reckless, high dose mammography experiments has increased breast cancer risks for the 400,000 women involved.

- Breast implants, particularly polyurethane foam, pose serious risks of breast cancer. Evidence on the carcinogenicity of polyurethane foam dates back to the early 1960's. One breakdown product of polyurethane is 2,4-toluenediamine which was removed from hair dyes in 1971 following discovery of its carcinogenicity. Frank admission of these risks are found in internal NCI, FDA and industry documents.

- The Tamoxifen "chemoprevention" trial is a travesty! Since 1992, the cancer establishment recruited 16,000 healthy women in a Tamoxifen "chemoprevention" trial. NCI and ACS claimed in their patient consent forms that Tamoxifen could substantially reduce breast cancer risks, while trivializing risks of drug complications. There is strong evidence of Tamoxifen's toxicity, including high risks of uterine, gastrointestinal and fatal liver cancer. "This trial is scientifically and ethically reckless, and participating institutions and clinicians are at serious risk of future malpractice claims," warned Dr. Epstein.

"The ICI/NBCAM public relations campaign has prevented women from knowing of avoidable causes of breast cancer," concluded Dr. Epstein.

October 18, 1995

NATIONAL MAMMOGRAPHY DAY

Commenting on tomorrow's National Mammography Day, Dr. Samuel Epstein, Chairman of the Cancer Prevention Coalition (CPC), charged that "this is a recklessly misleading and self-interested promotional event, more aptly named NATIONAL MAMMOSCAM DAY."

National Mammography Day, October 19, is the flagship of October's National Breast Cancer Awareness Month (NBCAM). NBCAM was conceived and funded in 1984 by Imperial Chemical Industries (ICI) and its U.S. subsidiary and spinoff Zeneca Pharmaceuticals. NBCAM is a multimillion-dollar deal with the cancer establishment, the National Cancer Institute (NCI) and American Cancer Society (ACS) and its multiple corporate sponsors, and the American College of Radiology.

ICI is one of the largest manufacturers of petrochemical and organochlorines, and Zeneca is the sole manufacturer of Tamoxifen, the world's top selling cancer drug widely used for breast cancer. Zeneca/ICI's financial sponsorship gives them control over every leaflet, poster, publication, and commercial produced by NBCAM.

ICI supports the NBCAM blame-the-victim theory of cancer causation, which attributes escalating rates of breast (and other) cancers to heredity and faulty lifestyle. This theory diverts attention away from avoidable exposures to carcinogenic industrial contaminants of air, water, food, consumer products, and the workplace—the same products which ICI has manufactured for decades. Ignoring prevention of breast cancer, NBCAM promotes "early" detection by mammography.

There are a wide range of serious problems with mammography, particularly with pre-menopausal women:

- There is no evidence of the effectiveness or benefit of mammography in pre-menopausal women.
- By the time breast cancers can be detected by mammography, they are up to 8 years old. By then, some will have spread to local lymph nodes or to distant organs, especially in younger women.
- Missed cancers (false negatives) are commonplace among younger women, as their dense breast tissues limit penetration by x-rays.
- About 1 in every 4 "tumors" identified by mammography in pre-menopausal women turns out not to be cancer following biopsy (false positive). Apart from needless anxiety, repeated surgery can

result in scarring, and delayed identification of early cancer that may subsequently develop.

- Regular mammography of younger women increases their cancer risks, particularly for women already at risk for familial reasons. Analysis of controlled trials over the last decade, has shown consistent increases in breast cancer mortality within a few years of commencing screening. This confirms evidence on the high sensitivity of the pre-menopausal breast, and on cumulative carcinogenic effects of radiation.

- Pre-menopausal women carrying the A-T gene, about 1.5 percent of women, are more radiation sensitive and at higher cancer risk from mammography. It has been estimated that up to 10,000 breast cancer cases each year are due to mammography of A-T carriers.

- Radiation, particularly from repeated pre-menopausal mammography, is likely to interact additively or synergistically with other avoidable causes of breast cancer, particularly estrogens (natural; medical; contaminants of meat from cattle feed additives; and estrogenic pesticides).

- Forceful compression of the breast during mammography, particularly in younger women, may cause the spread of small undetected cancers.

Pressured by this evidence on the ineffectiveness and risks of pre-menopausal mammography, NCI recently withdrew recommendations for such screening. This evidence is still ignored by NBCAM, supported by radiologists and giant mammography machine and film corporations, which has specifically targeted pre-menopausal women with high-pressured advertisements.

CPC urges the immediate phase-out of pre-menopausal mammography. Post-menopausal mammography should be restricted to major centers and exposure reduced to a minimum. Women should be provided with actual close measurements, rather than estimates. NCI and ACS should develop large-scale use of safe screening alternatives, including imaging techniques, and blood or urine tumor markers or immunologic tests.

A medical alert should be sent to women subjected to the Breast Cancer Detection Demonstration Project high dose radiation experiments commencing in 1972. These experiments were conducted in spite of explicit prior warnings by a National Academy of Sciences committee, and also by former senior NCI staffer, and noted epidemiologist, Dr. John Bailar. He cautioned, "Such radiation in pre-menopausal women would be likely to cause more breast cancers than could be detected." Dr. Bailar now concludes, "This experiment could well account for an "immediate investigation of the cancer establishment's reckless conduct by the President's Committee on Human Radiation Experiments."

April 1, 1998

CANCER REPORT CARD GETS A FAILING GRADE

At a highly publicized March 12, 1998, Washington, DC press briefing, the National Cancer Institute (NCI) and American Cancer Society (the cancer establishment), together with the Centers for Disease Control and Prevention, released a "Report Card" announcing the recent reversal of "an almost 20-year trend of increasing cancer cases and death," as detailed in the March 15 issue of the journal *Cancer*. "These numbers are the first proof that we are on the right track," enthused NCI director Dr. Richard Klausner. This news received extensive and uncritical nation-wide media coverage.

These claims were based on a comparison between NCI's published statistics for 1973-1990 and 1973-1995. However, the more recent information remains unpublished and, according to senior NCI statistician Dr. Lynn Ries, is still being analyzed. More importantly, a critical review of the *Cancer* publication is hardly reassuring. The claimed reversal in overall mortality rates is not only minimal but exaggerated. It is largely due to a reduction in lung cancer deaths from smoking in men, reflecting personal lifestyle choices, and to improved access to health care rather than to any improvements in treatment and survival rates. Additionally, any true decline would be considerably less if the mortality rates were appropriately based on the current age distribution of the U.S. population, rather than that of 1970, with its relatively higher representation of younger age groups, as misleadingly calculated by NCI. These criticisms are in general consistent with those detailed in a May 1997 *New England Journal of Medicine* article, "Cancer Undefeated," by former NCI epidemiologist Dr. John Bailar.

The claimed reversal in the incidence of cancers of "all sites" is minimal and statistically insignificant, as are similar claims for leukemia and prostate cancer. Even this minimal reduction of prostate cancer is highly questionable as admitted by Report Card authors: "The decreased incidence rates [of prostate cancer] may be the result of decreased utilization of PSA [prostate specific antigen] screening tests . . . during the early 1990's." While there were significant reductions in the incidence of lung, colon/rectum and bladder cancers, there were significant and sharp increases in uterine cancer, melanoma, and non-Hodgkin's lymphoma. Moreover, there was no decline in breast cancer rates, which remain unchanged at their current high level. Curiously, no reference at all was made to testicular cancer in young adults nor to childhood cancer, whose rates have dramatically increased in recent decades.

The Report Card apart, there are disturbing questions on the reliability of NCI's incidence statistics. This is well illustrated by wild reported variations since 1973 for the percent changes in the incidence of childhood cancer:

1973-1980	+21%
1973-1989	+10%
1973-1990	+1%
1973-1991	-8%
1973-1994	+31%

The Report Card's optimistic and misleading assurances, the latest in a series of smoke and mirror break-through since 1971 when President Nixon launched the "War Against Cancer," are designed to divert attention from the escalating incidence of cancer, which has reached epidemic proportions. Cancer now strikes 1 in 2 men and 1 in 3 women, up from an incidence of 1 in 4 a few decades ago. Meanwhile, our ability to treat and cure most cancer, apart from relatively infrequent cancers particularly those of children, remains virtually unchanged. The Report Card is also designed to neutralize criticism of NCI's intransigent fixation on diagnosis, treatment, and basic genetic research, coupled with indifference to prevention, which receives minimal priorities and resources—less than 5% of NCI's budget. Further illustrative is the fact that NCI has never testified before Congress or regulatory agencies on the substantial published evidence on the wide range of carcinogenic industrial contaminants of air, water, the workplace, and consumer products—food, household products, and cosmetics—and on the need to prevent such avoidable and involuntary exposures. Nor has NCI recognized the public's right-to-know of such critical information, which plays a major role in escalating cancer rates, nor have they developed community outreach prevention programs. Finally, the Report Card is designed to further buttress aggressive lobbying by the cancer establishment and cancer drug industry for a major increase in NCI's budget from the current $2.6 billion, up from $223 million in 1971, to the requested $3.2 billion in 1999.

Rather than increasing NCI's bloated budget, drastic reforms are needed to explicitly re-orient its mission and priorities to cancer causes and prevention.

August 25, 1998

THE CANCER DRUG INDUSTRY "MARCH" SERIOUSLY MISLEADS THE NATION

On September 25 and 26, the cancer drug industry will hold the "March," led by Gen. Norman Schwarzkopf, in Washington, D.C., and elsewhere in the nation, under a banner promising "Research Cures Cancer." Well-meaning but misled citizens will march for a seemingly important crusade which, in reality, promotes enormous profits for the pharmaceutical industry.

Funded with over $3 million by multibillion dollar cancer drug industries—including the global giants Bristol-Myers Squibb, Eli Lilly, Pharmacia & Upjohn—with support from main stream cancer survivor groups, the American Cancer Society (ACS) and, behind the scenes, the National Cancer Institute (NCI), the goal of the "March" is to mobilize grass roots backing for doubling NCI's current budget from $2.6 billion to over $5 billion by 2003.

This is déjà vu all over again. In a full-page December 9, 1969 New York Times advertisement entitled "MR. NIXON, YOU CAN CURE CANCER," paid for by the "Citizens' Committee for the Conquest of Cancer" whose leaders represented the cancer establishment, the public and government were exhorted: "We are so close to a cure for cancer. We lack only the will and the kind of money and comprehensive planning that went into putting a man on the moon.—Why don't we try to conquer cancer by America's 200th birthday." Responding to these misleading assurances, in December 1971, President Nixon was duped into declaring the "War Against Cancer" and sharply increasing NCI's budget.

Some $25 billion and 25 years later, there has been little if any significant improvement in treatment and survival rates for most common cancers despite contrary misleading hype by the cancer establishment and periodic claims for the latest miracle cancer drugs, claims which rarely have been substantiated. Meanwhile, the incidence of cancer, particularly non-smoking cancers, has escalated to epidemic proportions with lifetime cancer risks now approaching one in two.

The reason for losing the war against cancer is not a shortage of funds but their gross misallocation. NCI and ACS remain myopically fixated on damage control—diagnosis and treatment—and basic genetic research with, not always benign, indifference to cancer prevention. The establishment has trivialized escalating cancer rates and explained them away as due to faulty lifestyle, to the virtual exclusion of the major role of unwitting and avoidable exposures to industrial carcinogens in air, water, consumer products—food, cosmetics and toiletries, and household products—and the workplace. NCI and ACS have devoted the most minimal resources and priorities to research on such avoidable causes of cancer, failed to warn the public of these avoidable risks, and failed to provide Congress and regulatory agencies with available scientific information which would allow development of corrective legislative and regulatory action. Responding to recent criticisms, NCI has defensively claimed $1 billion expenditures for cancer prevention. However, more realistic estimates are well under $100 million, less than 3% of NCI's total budget.

Cancer establishment policies are strongly influenced by pervasive interlocking relationships and conflicts of interest with the cancer drug industry. With taxpayers' money, NCI funded the R & D for the anticancer drug Taxol manufactured by Bristol-Myers. Following completion of expensive clinical trials, the public paid further for developing the drug's manufacturing process. Once completed, NCI gave this industry exclusive right to sell Taxol at an inflationary price, about $5 per milligram, over 20 times the cost of production.

Taxol is not an isolated example. Taxpayers have funded NCI's R & D for over two-thirds of all cancer drugs now on the market. In a surprisingly frank admission, Samuel Broder, NCI director from 1989 to 1995, stated the obvious: "The NCI has become what amounts to a government pharmaceutical company." It should further be noted that the U.S. spends about five times more on chemotherapy per patient than Great Britain, although this is not matched by any difference in survival rates.

Not surprisingly, with enthusiastic support from the ACS, NCI has effectively blocked funding for research and clinical trials on promising non-toxic alternative cancer therapies in favor of highly toxic and largely ineffective patented drugs developed by the cancer drug industry. Additionally, the cancer establishment has systematically harassed the proponents of alternative cancer treatment.

These basic criticisms of cancer establishment policies and deceptive practices, with particular reference to minimal prevention priorities, were strongly endorsed in a February 1992 statement by a group of 65 leading national experts in public health and cancer prevention, including past directors of federal agencies, who urged drastic reforms of NCI policies and that funding for cancer prevention should be increased to equal that for all other NCI programs combined. This was followed in 1995 by a warning from 15 public interest organizations, representing some 5 million Americans, of the misleading industry-sponsored "Research Cures Cancer" campaign, and a recommendation that NCI be held accountable for its failed policies in losing the war against cancer.

Rather than increasing NCI's budget, it should be frozen and held hostage to urgent needs for drastic monitored reforms directed to major emphasis on cancer prevention rather than damage control. Furthermore, Congress should subject the cancer establishment/drug industry complex to detailed investigation and ongoing scrutiny.

October 26, 1999

AMERICAN CANCER SOCIETY INDICTED FOR LOSING THE WINNABLE WAR AGAINST CANCER

An article, "American Cancer Society: The World's Wealthiest 'Non-Profit' Institution," by Dr. Samuel Epstein, just published in the International Journal of Health Services, the leading international public health and policy journal, charges that the American Cancer Society (ACS) "is fixated on damage control . . . diagnosis and treatment . . . and basic molecular biology, with indifference or even hostility to cancer prevention." ACS also trivializes the escalating incidence of cancer which has reached epidemic proportions and makes grossly misleading claims on dramatic progress in the treatment and cure of cancer. This myopic mind-set and derelict policy is compounded by interlocking conflicts of interests with the cancer drug, agrichemical, and other industries. The following is illustrative:

- Since 1982, the ACS has adopted a highly restrictive policy insisting on unequivocal human evidence on carcinogenicity before taking any position on cancer risks. Accordingly, the ACS has actively campaigned against the 1958 Delaney law banning the deliberate addition to food of any amount of chemical additive shown to induce cancer, even in well-validated federal animal tests.
- In a joint 1992 statement with the Chlorine Institute, the ACS supported the continued use of organochlorine pesticides in spite of their recognized environmental persistence and carcinogenicity.
- In 1993, just before PBS Frontline aired the special entitled "In Our Children's Food," the ACS sent a memorandum in support of the pesticide industry to some 48 regional divisions which preemptively trivialized pesticides as a cause of childhood cancer and reassured the public that residues of carcinogenic pesticide in food are safe, even for babies.
- In Cancer Facts & Figures, the ACS annual publication designed to provide the public with "basic facts" on cancer, there is little or no mention of prevention. Examples include no mention of: dusting the genital area with talc as a known cause of ovarian cancer; parental exposure to occupational carcinogens, domestic use of pesticides, or frequent consumption of nitrite colored hot dogs (resultantly contaminated with carcinogenic nitrosamines) as major causes of childhood cancer; and prolonged use of oral contraceptives or hormonal replacement therapy as major causes of breast cancer. Fact & Figures,

1997, also misrepresented that "since women may not be able to alter their personal risk factors, the best opportunity for reducing mortality is early detection." This statement ignores overwhelming evidence on a wide range of ways by which women of all ages can reduce their risks of breast cancer, including regular use of the cheap non-prescription drug aspirin.

- The ACS, together with the National Cancer Institute, has strongly promoted the use of Tamoxifen, the world's top-selling cancer drug ($400 million annually) manufactured by Zeneca, for allegedly preventing breast cancer in healthy women, evidence for which is highly arguable at best. More seriously, ACS has trivialized the dangerous and sometimes lethal complications of Tamoxifen including blood clots, lung embolism, and aggressive uterine cancer, and fails to warn that the drug is a highly potent liver carcinogen.

Conflicts of interest are further reflected in the ACS Foundation Board of Trustees which includes corporate executives from the pharmaceutical, cancer drug, investment, and media industries. They include David R. Bethume, president of Lederle laboratories, Gordon Binder, CEO of Amgen (a leading biotech cancer drug company), and Sumner M. Redstone, chairman of the Board of Viacom, Inc.

Other concerns relate to the "non-profit status" of the ACS whose annual budget is some $500 million. Most funds raised go to pay high overhead, salaries fringe benefits, and travel expenses of national executives in Atlanta, CEO's who ear six-figure salaries in several states, and hundreds of other employees working in some 3000 regional offices. Less than 16% of all monies raised are spent on direct patient services; salaries and overhead for most ACS affiliates exceed 50%, although most direct community services are handled by unpaid volunteers. While ACS cash assets and reserves approach $1 billion, it continues to plead poverty and lament the lack of funds for cancer research. Not surprisingly and as reported in the Chronicle of Philanthropy, the leading U.S. charity watchdog, the ACS is "more interested in accumulating wealth than saving lives." It should further be noted that the ACS uses 10 employees and spends $1 million a year on direct lobbying, and is the only known charity that makes contributions to political parties.

Based on these considerations, the International Journal of Health Services article urged that, in the absence of drastic reforms, contributions to the ACS should be diverted to public interest and environmental group directly involved in cancer prevention. This is the only message that this "charity" can no longer ignore.

May 30, 2000

AMERICAN CANCER SOCIETY: LONG ON PROMISE, SHORT ON DELIVERY

The American Cancer Society (ACS) claims to be dedicated to "preventing cancer and saving lives—through research education, advocacy, and service." What could be more worthy objectives, especially in view of the escalating incidence of cancer, with lifetime cancer risks now reaching one in two men and one in three for women?

Unfortunately, the ACS fails to meet its objectives. Instead, the charity is accumulating great wealth, with $900 million reserves in cash, real estate and other assets. Most of its funds come from public donations of under $100. Additional funding is provided by bequests and high profile fundraising events, such as the springtime daffodil sale and relay races.

In 1998, the society spent about $150 million on "Supporting Services," overhead, salaries in the $300,000 range, benefits and travel for national executives in Atlanta, fundraising, and public relations. Typical ACS affiliates, which raise national funds, spend over half of their budgets on salaries, pensions, fringe benefits and overhead, with under 16 percent on direct community services, most of which are handled by unpaid volunteers. Meanwhile, five of the society's division executives received salaries of about $230,000.

As the ACS purse grows, its spending on research and other programs remains low. While the 1998 budget report gives the clear impression that generous resources are allocated to its four "Program Services," they receive under 50 percent of its budget, as follows: "Research on the causes, cure and prevention of cancer," $91 million; "Prevention programs that provide the public and professionals with information on how to reduce risks of developing cancer," $80 million; "Detection/Treatment" programs, $59 million; and "Patient Services" programs, $77 million.

Responding to recent well-documented criticism of not always benign indifference to cancer prevention, the ACS claims that it funded 19 large research grants in 1998 on "Environmental Carcinogenesis" at a cost of $2.6 million. However, only two grants funded for $330,000, could reasonably qualify as environmental cancer research, while virtually all other were in the unrelated field of molecular biology. The ACS also claims that it funded 92 "Prevention" grants with $23 million, while these also largely dealt with molecular biology research. Tobacco related programs accounted for only $1.3 million, while research on diet per se, excluding any consideration of contamination with carcinogenic pesticides, accounted for $1.1 million. In fact, analysis of its $2.6 million carcinogenesis programs reveals that expenditures on environmental, occupational, and industrial causes of cancer totaled $1 million, well under 1 percent of its annual budget.

More than anything else, the society seems scared of becoming just another face in the crowd of cancer interests in Washington. Thus, in 1998, Linda Hay Crawford, then vice president for governmental relations, admitted to the Associated Press that the society had used 10 employees for direct lobbying at costs approaching $1 million. "Lobbying" also including $30,000 donations, equitably balanced between Democratic and Republican governor's associations. "We wanted to look like players and be players," Crawford explained to AP.

This practice, however, has been sharply challenged. The AP story quoted the national Charities Information Bureau as stating that it "does not know of any other charity that makes contributions to political parties." The director of the IRS Exempt Organization Division, Marcus Owens, warned that: "The bottom line is, campaign contributions will jeopardize a charity's exempt status." Other troubling misallocations on the national political scene include hiring public relations firms that also represent tobacco clients. Recently, the society had to discontinue its association with two such firms: Shandwick International and Edelman Public Relations.

In an effort to dominate the national cancer agenda, nearly two years ago, ACS recruited former President George Bush to run a curious political structure called the National Dialogue on Cancer. This was recently followed by a related closed door ACS initiative to rewrite the 1971 National Cancer Act by an "Independent Advisory Committee," sponsored by Senator Dianne Feinstein (D-Calif.). Shunned by many major patient advocacy groups, the National Cancer Institute and professional oncologists, and with strong protests by cancer prevention groups, the future of the ACS-Feinstein initiative, seems questionable. More pointedly, John Durant, former executive vice president of the American Society for Clinical Oncology, charged in the January 21, 2000 *Cancer Letter*, a respected trade publication, that the underlying motivation for these initiatives "was an issue of control by the ACS over the cancer agenda. They are protecting their fundraising capacity."

Based on an analysis of ACS budgets and programs, *The Chronicle of Philanthropy*, the leading charity watchdog, published a statement that the ACS is "more interested in accumulating wealth than saving lives." Donors wanting to make contributions to a worthy cancer charity should think twice before selecting the ACS.

June 12, 2001

THE AMERICAN CANCER SOCIETY IS THREATENING THE NATIONAL CANCER PROGRAM

Operating behind closed doors and with powerful political connections, Dr. Samuel Epstein, charges the American Cancer Society (ACS) with forging a questionably legal alliance with the federal Centers for Disease Control and Prevention (CDC) in attempts to hijack the National Cancer Program. The ACS is also charged with virtual neglect of cancer prevention.

Dr. Quentin Young, warns: "The ACS political agenda reveals a pattern of self interest, conflicts of interest, lack of accountability and non-transparency to all of which the media have responded with deafening silence."

Among their concerns:

- The National Cancer Act, the cornerstone of the National Cancer Institute's (NCI) war on cancer, is under powerful attack by the ACS, the world's largest non-religious "charity." The plan was hatched in September 1998 when, meeting behind closed doors, the ACS created a "National Dialogue on Cancer" (NDC), co-chaired by former President Bush and Barbara Bush, with representatives from the CDC, the giant cancer drug industry, and Collaborating Partners from survivor advocacy groups. The NDC leadership then unilaterally spun off a National Cancer Legislative Committee, co-chaired by Dr. John Seffrin, CEO of the ACS and Dr. Vincent DeVita, Director of the Yale Cancer Center and former NCI Director, to advise Congress on re-writing the National Cancer Act.
- The relationships between the ACS, NDC and its Legislative Committee raise questions on conflicts of interest. John Durant, former executive president of the American Society for Clinical Oncology, charged: "It has always seemed to me that this was an issue of control by the ACS over the cancer agenda—. They are protecting their own fundraising capacity" from competition by survivor groups.
- The ACS-CDC relationship is focused on diverting political emphasis and funds away from NCI's peer-reviewed scientific research to CDC's community programs, which center on community screening, behavioral intervention, and tobacco cessation rather than prevention.
- There are major concerns on interlocking ACS-CDC interests. CDC has improperly funded ACS with a $3 million sole source four-year cooperative agreement. In turn, ACS has made strong efforts to upgrade CDC's role in the National Cancer Program, increase appropriations

for CDC's non-peer reviewed programs, and facilitate its access to tobacco litigation money.

- The ACS priority for tobacco cessation programs is inconsistent with its strong ties to the industry. Shandwick International, representing R.J. Reynolds, and Edelman, representing Brown & Williamson Tobacco Company, have been major PR firms for the NDC and its Legislative Committee.

- ACS has made questionably legal contributions to Democratic and Republican Governors' Associations. "We wanted to look like players and be players," ACS explained.

- DeVita, the Legislative Committee co-chair, is also chairman of the Medical Advisory Board of CancerSource.com, a website launched by Jones & Bartlett which publishes the ACS Consumer's Guide to Cancer Drugs; three other members of the Committee also serve on the board. DeVita thus appears to be developing his business interests in a publicly-funded forum.

- The ACS has a longstanding track record of indifference and even hostility to cancer prevention. This is particularly disturbing in view of the escalating incidence of cancer now striking one in two men and one in three women in their lifetimes. Recent examples include issuing a joint statement with the Chlorine Institute justifying the continued global use of persistent organochlorine pesticides, and also supporting the industry in trivializing dietary pesticide residues as avoidable risks of childhood cancer. ACS policies are further exemplified by allocating under 0.1 percent of its $700 million annual budget to environmental and occupational causes of cancer.

These considerations clearly disqualify the ACS from any leadership role in the National Cancer Program. The public should be encouraged to redirect funding away from the ACS to cancer prevention advocacy groups. ACS conduct, particularly its political lobbying and relationship to CDC, should be investigated by Congressional Appropriations and Oversight committees. These committees should also recommend that the National Cancer Program direct the highest priority to cancer prevention.

ENDORSER:

Quentin D. Young, MD
Chairman of the Health and Medicine Policy Research Group
Past President of American Public Health Association
Chicago, Illinois

May 9, 2002

ESCALATING INCIDENCE OF CHILDHOOD CANCER IS IGNORED BY THE NATIONAL CANCER INSTITUTE AND AMERICAN CANCER SOCIETY

Since passage of the 1971 National Cancer Act, launching the "War Against Cancer," the incidence of childhood cancer has steadily escalated to alarming levels. Childhood cancers have increased by 26% overall, while the incidence of particular cancers has increased still more: acute lymphocytic leukemia, 62%; brain cancer, 50%; and bone cancer, 40%. The federal National Cancer Institute (NCI) and the "charitable" American Cancer Society (ACS), the cancer establishment, have failed to inform the public, let alone Congress and regulatory agencies, of this alarming information. As importantly, they have failed to publicize well-documented scientific information on avoidable causes responsible for the increased incidence of childhood cancer. Examples include:

- Over 20 U.S. and international studies have incriminated paternal and maternal exposures (pre-conception, during conception and post-conception) to a wide range of occupational carcinogens as major causes of childhood cancer.
- There is substantial evidence on the risks of brain cancer and leukemia in children from frequent consumption of nitrite-dyed hot dogs; consumption during pregnancy has been similarly incriminated. Nitrites, added to meat for coloring purposes, have been shown to react with natural chemicals in meat (amines) to form a potent carcinogenic nitrosamine.
- Consumption of non-organic fruits and vegetables, particularly in baby food, contaminated with high concentrations of multiple residues of carcinogenic pesticides, poses major risks of childhood cancer, besides delayed cancers in adult life.
- Numerous studies have shown strong associations between childhood cancers, particularly brain cancer, non-Hodgkin's lymphoma and leukemia, and domestic exposure to pesticides from uses in the home, including pet flea collars, lawn and garden; another major source of exposure is commonplace use in schools.
- Use of lindane, a potent carcinogen in shampoos for treating lice and scabies, infesting about six million children annually, is associated with major risks of brain cancer; lindane is readily absorbed through the skin.

- Treatment of children with Ritalin for "Attention Deficit Disorders" poses risks of cancer, in the absence of informed parental consent. Ritalin has been shown to induce highly aggressive rare liver cancers in rodents at doses comparable to those prescribed to children.
- Maternal exposure to ionizing radiation, especially in late pregnancy, is strongly associated with excess risks of childhood leukemia.

It is of particular significance that the cancer establishment ignored the continuing increase in the incidence of childhood cancer in its heavily promoted, but highly arguable, March 1998 "claim to have reversed an almost 20-year trend of increasing cancer cases."

The failure of the cancer establishment to warn of these avoidable cancer risks reflects mind-sets fixated on damage control—screening, diagnosis, and treatment—and basic genetic research, with indifference to primary prevention, as defined by research and public education on avoidable causes of cancer. For the ACS, this indifference extends to a well-documented long-standing track record of hostility, such as supporting the Chlorine Institute in defending the continued global use of chlorinated organic pesticides, and Assurances in the 2002 Cancer Facts and Figures that cancer risks from dietary Pesticides and ionizing radiation are all at such low levels as to be "negligible." This indifference to primary prevention is compounded by conflicts of interest, particularly with the giant cancer drug industry. Not surprisingly, The Chronicle of Philanthropy, the nation's leading charity watchdog, published a statement that: "The ACS is more interested in accumulating wealth than saving lives."

The minimal priorities of the cancer establishment for prevention reflects mind-sets and policies and not lack of resources. NCI's annual budget has increased some 20-fold since passage of the 1971 Act, from $220 million to $4.2 billion, while revenues of the ACS are now about $800 million. NCI expenditures on primary prevention have been estimated as under 4% of its budget, while ACS allocates less than 0.1% of its revenues to primary prevention and "environmental carcinogenesis."

It should be particularly stressed that fetuses, infants and children are much more vulnerable and sensitive to toxic and carcinogenic exposures than are adults. It should also be recognized that the majority of carcinogens also induce other chronic toxic effects, especially in fetuses, infants and children. These include endocrine disruptive and reproductive, hematological, immunological and genetic, for which there are no available incidence trend data comparable to those for cancer.

The continued silence of the cancer establishment on avoidable causes of childhood, besides a wide range of other, cancers is in flagrant denial of the specific charge of the 1971 National Cancer Act "to disseminate cancer information to the public." As seriously, this silence is a denial of the public's inalienable democratic right-to-know of information directly impacting on their health and lives, and of their right to influence public policy.

Whether against cancer or terrorism, war is best fought by preemptive strategies based on prevention rather than reactively on damage control. As importantly, the war against cancer must be waged by leadership accountable to the public interest and not, as is still the case, special agenda private interests. The time for open public debate on national cancer policy is long overdue.

ENDORSER:

Quentin D. Young, MD
Chairman of the Health and Medicine Policy Research Group
Past President of American Public Health Association
Chicago, Illinois

February 25, 2003

NATIONAL CANCER INSTITUTE LEADERSHIP IS OUT OF TOUCH WITH REALITY

In a speech to an advisory board, the Director of the National Cancer Institute (NCI) pledged to eliminate "the suffering and death" from cancer by 2015.

NCI Director Andrew von Eschenbach in a Feb. 11 speech to the National Cancer Advisory Board stated: "I have set out . . . a challenge goal that shapes our mission and shapes our vision . . . to eliminate the suffering and death due to cancer, and to do it by 2015."

Dr. von Eschenbach's goal is irresponsible and unrealistic, said Samuel S. Epstein, M.D., Chairman of the Cancer Prevention Coalition. "What is the possible scientific basis for such claims?" Epstein asked. "Does Dr. von Eschenbach know something no one else knows? Is he familiar with the NCI data on incidence and mortality? What great advances or breakthroughs does he know, of which no one else is aware? Has he been talking with God?"

Since 1971, the overall incidence of cancer has escalated to epidemic proportions, now striking about 1.3 million and killing about 550,000 annually; nearly one in two men and more than one in three women now develop cancer in their lifetimes. While smoking is unquestionably the single largest cause of cancer, the incidence of lung cancer in men has declined sharply. In striking contrast, there have been major increases in the incidence of a wide range of non-smoking cancers in men and women, and also of childhood cancers.

The current cancer epidemic does not reflect lack of resources. Paradoxically, NCI's escalating budget is paralleled by the escalating incidence of cancer. Since 1971, NCI's budget has increased approximately 30-fold, from $220 million to $4.6 billion.

According to the Cancer Prevention Coalition, the fundamental reason why we are losing the winnable war against cancer is because NCI's mind-set is fixated on damage control-screening, diagnosis, and treatment-and basic research. This is coupled with indifference to preventing a wide range of avoidable exposures to industrial carcinogens, contaminating the totality of the environment—air, water, and soil—the workplace, and consumer products—food, cosmetics and toiletries and household products. This denial of the public's right-to-know of such avoidable cancer risks is in contrast to NCI's stream of press releases, briefings, and media reports claiming the latest advances in treatment and basic research.

The silence of the NCI, besides the American Cancer Society (ACS), on avoidable causes of cancer has tacitly encouraged corporate polluters and industries to continue manufacturing and marketing carcinogenic products. This silence also violates amendments of the National Cancer Act, calling for "an expanded and intensified research program for the prevention of cancer caused by occupational or environmental exposure to carcinogens."

Nevertheless, NCI's prevention policies are virtually restricted to faulty lifestyle considerations. As strikingly exemplified in von Eschenbach's recent speech, prevention is defined only in terms of tobacco, "energy balance" and obesity. However, this is hardly surprising as von Eschenbach was President-Elect of the ACS prior to his appointment as NCI Director. The ACS Cancer Facts and Figures 2002 dismissively reassures that carcinogenic exposures from dietary pesticides, "toxic wastes in dump sites," ionizing radiation from "closely controlled" nuclear power plants, and non-ionizing radiation, are all "at such low levels that risks are negligible."

Dr. von Eschenbach also remains Director of the ACS 1998 National Dialogue on Cancer, which seeks a major role in federal cancer policies. It may be further noted that The Chronicle of Philanthropy, the nation's leading charity watch dog, has published a statement that the ACS "is more interested in accumulating wealth than saving lives."

These concerns are detailed in the Cancer Prevention Coalition (CPC) report, "Stop Cancer Before It Starts Campaign: How to Win the Losing War Against Cancer," released at a Feb. 20 Washington, D.C., press conference. This report is endorsed by some 100 leading cancer prevention scientists, public health and policy experts, and representatives of concerned citizen groups, who advocate major reforms of national cancer policies.

May 23, 2003

THE AMERICAN CANCER SOCIETY MISLEADS THE PUBLIC IN THE MAY 26 DISCOVERY HEALTH CHANNEL PROGRAM

In a one-hour special on the "TOP 10 CANCER MYTHS," the American Cancer Society (ACS) claims to set the record straight. However, these claims are seriously flawed.

While admitting that number of people diagnosed with cancer is increasing, the ACS explains this away as due to aging of the population, and the frequency of cancer in the elderly. However, federal statistics adjusted for aging show a 24% increased incidence rate over the last three decades. What's more, most major increases have involved non-smoking related cancers. These cancers include: non-Hodgkin's lymphoma, 87%; thyroid, 71%; testis, 67%; post-menopausal breast, 54%; and brain, 28%. More disturbing is the escalating incidence of childhood cancers: acute lymphocytic leukemia, 62%; brain, 50%; bone, 40%; and kidney, 14%. Of related interest is an analysis of leading causes of death from 1973 to 1999. Cancer has increased by 30%, while mortality from heart disease decreased by 21%.

Worse still, the ACS has failed to inform the public about scientifically well-documented causes of a wide range of non-smoking related cancers. The ACS goes further by dismissing evidence on risks from domestic use of pesticides, although several studies have clearly shown a strong relationship with childhood cancers. In its recommendation for high vegetable, fruit, and grain diets, ACS ignores the fact that these, including baby foods, are highly contaminated with carcinogenic pesticides, while ignoring the availability of safe organic products. The ACS goes even further in dismissing such concerns. In its Cancer Facts and Figures 2002, ACS reassured that cancer risks from dietary pesticides, besides hazardous waste sites, and ionizing radiation from "closely controlled" nuclear plants, are at such low levels as to be "negligible."

The CANCER MYTHS are consistent with its long-standing track record on prevention, policies, and conflicts of interest. In 1978, the ACS refused a Congressional request to support the Clean Air Act. In 1992, the ACS supported the Chlorine Institute by defending the continued use of carcinogenic chlorinated pesticides. In 1993, just before PBS aired the Frontline special, "In Our Children's Food," the ACS came out in support of the pesticide industry. In a damage—control memorandum, sent to some 48 regional divisions and their 3,000 local offices, the ACS trivialized pesticides as a cause of childhood cancer. ACS also reassured the public that food contaminated with carcinogenic pesticides is safe, even for babies.

In 1994, the ACS published a highly flawed study designed to reassure women on the safety of dark permanent hair dyes, and to trivialize the risks of non-Hodgkin's lymphoma, breast, and other cancers as documented in over six prior reports.

Analysis of the 1998 ACS budget revealed that it allocated less than 0.1% of its $700 million revenues to "Environmental Carcinogenesis."

In 2000, it was discovered that the ACS had close ties to PR firms for the tobacco industry—Shandwick International, representing R.J. Reynolds Holdings, and Edelman, representing Brown & Williamson Tobacco Company. These firms were promptly dismissed once the embarrassing news leaked out.

This indifference or hostility of the ACS to cancer prevention is less surprising in view of its pervasive conflicts of interest with the cancer drug, petrochemical, cosmetics, power plants, and other industries.

Not surprisingly, the authoritative U.S. charity watchdog, The Chronicle of Philanthropy, has warned against the transfer of money from the public purse to private hands. "The ACS is more interested in accumulating wealth than in saving lives."

February 23, 2004

SPINNING THE LOSING CANCER WAR

In politics, spinning is an art form. Most accept spinning as a fact of life, whether choosing a politician or merely a bar of soap. However, few would accept this gamesmanship for life and death issues of cancer, particularly if the spinning is underwritten by taxpayers.

But, when it comes to the cancer war, the Pollyannaish promises of the federal National Cancer Institute (NCI) and the non-profit American Cancer Society (ACS) are no more reliable than political flack.

Recent headlines in national newspapers, based on NCI and ACS assurances, report that the "Rate of Cancer Deaths Continues to Drop." This reinforces longstanding claims of miracle "breakthrough" treatments, that mortality would be halved by 2000, that the nation had "turned the corner" in the cancer war, and that "considerable progress has been made in reducing the burden of cancer." However, these claims don't even pass the laugh test.

Cancer death rates have remained unchanged since President Nixon declared the 1971 War Against Cancer. Nearly one in two men, and more than one in three women are now struck by cancer. Cancer has become a disease of "mass destruction."

Contrary to the NCI and ACS, the current cancer epidemic is not due to faulty lifestyle-smoking, unhealthy diet, and obesity. American men smoke less today, and lung cancer rates are steadily dropping. In striking contrast, the incidence of environmentally, and non-smoking related cancers has escalated sharply: non-Hodgkin's lymphoma by 71 percent, testes and thyroid cancers by 54 percent each, post-menopausal breast cancer by 37 percent, and myeloid leukemia by 15 percent; various childhood cancers have increased from 20 to 60 percent. For African Americans, the news is worse: incidence rates have increased by up to 120 percent.

The escalating incidence of non-smoking adult cancers and childhood cancers is paralleled by the 30-fold increase in NCI's budget from $220 million in 1972 to the current $4.6 billion. The ACS budget has increased from $130 to $800 million, with about $1 billion in reserves. It seems that the more we spend on cancer, the more cancer we get.

The reason we are losing this winnable war is because NCI and ACS priorities remain fixated on damage control—screening, diagnosis, and treatment—and related basic research. All merit substantial funding. However, less funding would be needed if more cancer was prevented, with less to treat.

Responding to criticisms of such imbalanced priorities, NCI now allocates 12% of its budget to "prevention and control," and requires its nationwide

Centers to have a "prevention component." However, cancer prevention continues to be narrowly defined in terms of faulty lifestyle, and screening, and excludes any reference to avoidable causes of cancer from exposures to industrial carcinogens. These include: contaminants of air, water, food, and the workplace; ingredients in cosmetics and toiletries, and household products, particularly pesticides.

NCI's indifference to such avoidable causes of cancer extends to denial. For example, NCI claims that, "The causes of childhood cancer are largely unknown," in spite of substantial contrary evidence. Similarly, ACS reassures that carcinogenic exposures from dietary pesticides, "toxic wastes in dump sites," and radiation from "closely controlled" nuclear power plants are all "at such low levels that risks are negligible."

Not surprisingly, Congressman John Conyers (D-MI), Ranking Member of the House Judiciary Committee and Dean of the Congressional Black Caucus, recently warned that so much cancer carnage is preventable. "Preventable, that is if the NCI gets off the dime and does its job."

NCI and ACS policies are compounded by conflicts of interest, particularly with the cancer drug industry. In a 1998 Washington Post interview, Dr. Samuel Broder, NCI's former Director, dropped a bombshell: "The NCI has become what amounts to a government pharmaceutical company." Broder resigned from the NCI to become successive Chief Officer of two major cancer drugs companies.

The ACS has a fund raising apparatus which would make any Presidential candidate blush. Apart from public donations, the ACS swims in the largesse of over 300 Excalibur industry donors, each contributing over $100,000 annually. These include over 25 drug and biotech companies, and petrochemical and oil industries. Unbelievably, ACS legislative initiatives are handled by Edelman PR, the major lobbyist of the tobacco industry, and fast food and beverage companies, now targeted by anti-obesity litigation.

Not surprisingly, *The Chronicle of Philanthropy*, the nation's leading charity watchdog, has published a statement: "The ACS is more interested in accumulating wealth than saving lives."

The cancer war is certainly winnable, given radical changes in its high command and priorities, and given information on avoidable industrial causes of cancer is provided to the public and Congress. The President has finally conceded the need for an independent commission to investigate misrepresentations that led us into the war on Iraq. We should use a similar commission to investigate the much more lethal failure of the cancer war.

February 28, 2005

TIME TO PROTECT BABIES FROM DANGEROUS PRODUCTS

From shortly after birth, mothers tenderly wash and pamper their infants with a wide range of baby products. These include soaps, shampoos, lotions, and dusting powders, some of which are used several times daily.

However, how would mothers react if they discovered that these baby products contain a witch's brew of dangerous ingredients? Hopping mad could be a reasonable understatement.

Most disturbing are three groups of widely used ingredients known as "hidden carcinogens"—ingredients which are contaminated by carcinogens, or which break down to release carcinogens, or which are precursors of carcinogens—to which infants are about 100 times more sensitive than adults.

The largest group of hidden carcinogens includes dozens of wetting agents or detergents, particularly PEGs, Laureths, and Cetearemths, all of which are contaminated with the potent and volatile carcinogens ethylene oxide and dioxane. These carcinogens could readily be stripped off during ingredient manufacture, if the industry just made the effort to do so. Another hidden carcinogenic ingredient is lanolin, derived from sheep's wool, most samples of which are contaminated with DDT-like pesticides.

The second group includes another detergent, Triethanolamine (TEA) which, following interaction with nitrite, is a precursor of a highly potent nitrosamine carcinogen.

The third group includes Quaterniums and Diazolidinyl urea preservatives which break down in the product or skin to release the carcinogenic formaldehyde.

Of additional concern is another group of common preservatives, known as Parabens. Numerous studies over the last decade have shown that these are weakly estrogenic. They produce abnormal hormonal effects following application to the skin of infant rodents, particularly male, resulting in decreased testosterone levels, and urogenital abnormalities. Parabens have also been found to accumulate in the breasts of women with breast cancer.

The common use of Talc dusting powder can result in its inhalation, resulting in acute or chronic lung irritation and disease (talcosis), and even death. Additionally, Talc is a suspect cause of lung cancer, based on rodent tests.

Fragrances, containing numerous ingredients, are commonly used in baby products for the mother's benefit. However, over 25 of these ingredients are known to cause allergic dermatitis.

A final ingredient of particular concern is the harshly irritant sodium lauryl sulfate. A single application to adult human skin has been shown to damage its microscopic structure, increasing the penetration of carcinogenic and other toxic ingredients.

Most disturbing is the ready availability of safe alternatives for all these dangerous ingredients (long-standing information on which is detailed on the Cancer Prevention Coalition website, http://www.preventcancer.com). So, why is it that the multibillion-dollar cosmetic and toiletry industry has not acted on this information? The answer is that the major priority of the industry's trade association is "to protect the freedom of the industry to compete in a fair market place." At the same time, the association pursues a highly aggressive agenda against what it claims are "unreasonable or unnecessary labeling or warning requirements." As Senator Edward M. Kennedy (D.MA) stated at 1997 Hearings on the FDA Reform bill: "The cosmetics industry has borrowed a page from the playbook of the tobacco industry by putting profits ahead of public health."

Astoundingly, the interests of industry remain reinforced by the regulatory abdication of the Food and Drug Administration (FDA), in spite of its authority under the 1938 Federal Food, Drug and Cosmetics (FD&C) Act. Clearly, the FDA is the lap dog, rather than the watchdog, of the industry.

Of even greater concern is the reckless failure of the federal National Cancer Institute and the "non-profit" American Cancer Society to inform the public of the avoidable risks of cancer from the use of baby products, especially in view of the escalating incidence of childhood cancers over recent decades. However, the silence of the American Cancer Society is consistent with its over $100,000 annual funding from about a dozen major cosmetic and toiletry industries.

The protracted failure of Congress to enforce FDA's compliance with the FD&C Act has evoked the growing concern of State legislatures. Assemblywoman Judy Chu (D-Monterey Park) of the California Senate Health Committee, recently introduced landmark legislation that requires disclosure of all carcinogenic, hormonal, and otherwise toxic ingredients in cosmetics. Strongly backed by a coalition of consumer, women, occupational, and church groups, but opposed by powerful mainstream industry interests, the Bill failed to pass. However, this shot over the bows of the reckless mainstream industry marks the beginning of nationwide State initiatives to protect consumers and their babies from undisclosed dangerous products and ingredients. Safe alternative products and ingredients, including organic, are becoming increasingly available from non-mainstream companies.

ENDORSER:

Ronnie Cummins
National Director
Organic Consumers Association

October 28, 2005

THE LOOK GOOD . . . FEEL BETTER PROGRAM: BUT AT WHAT RISK?

Launched in 1989 by the Cosmetic, Toiletry, and Fragrance Association (CTFA) and the National Cosmetology Association, the Look Good . . . Feel Better Program is "dedicated to teaching women cancer patients beauty techniques to help restore their appearance and self-image during cancer treatment." About 30,000 breast and other cancer patients participate yearly, each receiving a free makeover and bag of makeup.

Just what could be more noble? Or so it might just seem. The Look Good Program is supported by 22 CTFA-member cosmetic companies, including multibillion-dollar household name global giants. Each year, member companies "donate over one million individual cosmetic and personal care products, valued at $10 million, and raise more than $2 million." The Program is administered nationwide by the American Cancer Society (ACS), "which manages volunteer training, and serves as the primary source of information to the public."

There is no doubt that the products donated by the cosmetic companies, such as eye and cheek colors, lipsticks, moisture lotions, pressed powders and other makeups, are restorative. However, there is also no doubt that the ACS and the companies involved are oblivious to or strangely silent on the dangers of the Look Good products, whose ingredients are readily absorbed through the skin.

A review of 12 Look Good products, marketed by six companies, reveals that 10 contain dangerous chemical ingredients. Based on longstanding scientific evidence, these pose risks of cancer, and also hormonal (endocrine disruptive) effects.

Evidence for the cancer risks is based on standard tests in rodents, and on human (epidemiological) studies. Evidence for the hormonal risks is based on test-tube tests with breast cancer cells, or by stimulating premature sexual development in infant rodents. Unbelievably, the ACS explicitly warns women undergoing chemotherapy—"Don't use hormonal creams."

Take for example Estee Lauder's LightSource Transforming Moisture Lotion, Chanel's Sheer Lipstick, and Merle Norman Eye Color. These products contain ingredients which are carcinogenic, contaminated with carcinogens, or precursors of carcinogens. The products also contain hormonal ingredients, known as parabens, one of which has been identified in breast cancer tissue, and incriminated as a probable cause of breast cancer.

The ACS silence with regard to the risks of the Look Good products extends more widely to cosmetics and personal care products used by women, personal care products used by men, and baby lotions and shampoos. This silence is also consistent with the imbalanced objectives of the ACS highly publicized annual "Breast Cancer Awareness Month." While dedicated to the early detection of breast cancer, this event is silent on a wide range of its avoidable causes, besides the escalating incidence of post-menopausal breast cancer, by nearly 40%, over the last three decades.

Of likely relevance to the ACS silence is its interlocking interests with the cosmetic, besides other industries. The major Look Good companies are among some 350 ACS "Excalibur Donors," each donating a minimum of $10,000 annually. Other donors include petrochemical, power plant, and hazardous waste industries, whose environmental pollutants have been incriminated as causes of breast, besides other, cancers. Not surprisingly, The Chronicle of Philanthropy, the nation's leading charity watchdog, has published a statement that "The ACS is more interested in accumulating wealth than saving lives."

The ACS silence is also shared by the National Cancer Institute (NCI), which is required by the 1971 National Cancer Act to provide the public with information on avoidable causes of cancer. In spite of $50 billion taxpayers funding since 1971, the NCI has joined with the ACS in denying the public's right to know of avoidable causes of cancer from industrial chemicals, radiation, and common prescription drugs. Both the NCI and ACS are locked at the hip in policies fixated on damage control-screening, diagnosis, treatment and treatment-related research-with indifference to cancer prevention due to avoidable exposures to chemical carcinogens in cosmetics, other consumer products, air and water.

Equally asleep at the wheel remains the Food and Drug Administration in spite of its explicit regulatory authority. The 1938 Federal Food, Drug and Cosmetic Act explicitly requires that "The label of cosmetic products shall bear a warning statement . . . to prevent a health hazard that may be associated with a product."

No wonder the nation is losing the winnable war against cancer.

October 16, 2007

BREAST CANCER AWARENESS MONTH MISLEADS WOMEN

In 1984, the American Cancer Society (ACS) inaugurated the National Breast Cancer Awareness Month (NBCAM), with its Oct. 17 flagship National Mammography Day. The NBCAM was conceived and funded by the Imperial Chemical Industries, a leading international manufacturer of petrochemicals, and its U.S. subsidiary Zeneca Pharmaceuticals. Zeneca is the sole manufacturer of Tamoxifen, claimed to reduce risks of breast cancer, even though it is toxic and carcinogenic.

The NBCAM assures premenopausal women that "early (mammography) detection results in a cure nearly 100 percent of the time." More specifically, the NBCAM is primarily directed to claims for reducing the incidence and mortality of breast cancer through early detection by annual mammography starting at age 40.

Still unrecognized by the ACS, and the National Cancer Institute (NCI), there is strong evidence that routine premenopausal mammography poses significant risks of breast cancer. The routine practice of taking four films annually for each breast results in approximately 1 rad (radiation absorbed dose) exposure, approximately 1,000 times greater than the dose from a single chest X-ray. Each rad exposure increases risks of breast cancer by about one percent, with a cumulative 10 percent increased risk for each breast over a decade's screening. Moreover, the premenopausal breast is highly sensitive to radiation. Not surprisingly, premenopausal mammography screening is practiced by no nation other than the U.S.

Risks of premenopausal mammography are some four-fold greater for the one to two percent of women who are carriers of the A-T gene (ataxia telangiectasia), and highly sensitive to the carcinogenic effects of radiation. By some estimates, this accounts for up to 20 percent of all breast cancers diagnosed annually.

Compounding these problems, missed cancers are common in premenopausal women due to the density of their breasts.

That most breast cancers are first recognized by women was admitted in 1985 by the ACS. "We must keep in mind that at least 90 percent of the women who develop breast cancer discover the tumors themselves." Furthermore, an analysis of several 1993 studies showed that women who regularly performed breast self-examination (BSE) detected their cancers much earlier than women failing to examine themselves. However, the effectiveness of BSE depends on training by skilled professionals, enhanced by annual clinical breast examination by a professional. In spite of such evidence, the ACS and radiologists dismiss BSE, and claim that "no studies have clearly shown the benefit of using BSE."

A leading Massachusetts newspaper featured a photograph of two women in their twenties in an ACS advertisement that promised early detection by mammography results in a cure "nearly 100 percent of the time." An ACS communications director, questioned by journalist Kate Dempsey, responded in an article published in the Massachusetts Women's Community's journal Cancer "The ad isn't based on a study. When you make an advertisement, you just say what you can to get women in the door. You exaggerate a point . . . Mammography today is a lucrative [and] highly competitive business." She just couldn't be any more correct.

With this background, it is not surprising that the NBCAM has neglected to inform women how they can reduce their risks of breast cancer. In fact, we know a great deal about its avoidable causes which are still trivialized or ignored by the ACS. These include:

- Prolonged use of the Pill, and estrogen replacement therapy.
- High consumption of meat which is heavily contaminated with potent natural or synthetic estrogens, or other sex hormones. These are recklessly implanted in cattle in feedlots prior to slaughter to increase muscle mass and profitability.
- Prolonged consumption of milk from cows injected with a genetically engineered growth hormone (rBGH) to increase milk production. This milk is contaminated with high levels of a natural growth factor, which increases risks of breast cancer by up to seven-fold.
- Prolonged exposure to a wide range of unlabeled hormonal ingredients in most cosmetics and personal care products.
- Living near hazardous waste sites, petrochemical plants, power lines, and nuclear plants.
- Occupational exposures of over one million women to carcinogens. These include benzene, ethylene oxide, methylene chloride, phenylenediamine hair dyes, and agricultural pesticides, including DDT residues.

ENDORSER:

Rosalie Bertell, PhD
Former President of the International Institute of Concern for Public Health, Toronto, Canada
Regent of the International Physicians for Humanitarian Medicine, Geneva, Switzerland

July 22, 2009

SAFE BREAST SELF EXAM BY YOUNG WOMEN VS. DANGERS OF MAMMOGRAPHY

Critics of a Bill promoting training secondary school students to do breast self examinations to detect cancer are ignoring the risks of premenopausal mammography.

On March 26 this year, Representatives Debbie Wasserman-Schultz (D-FL) and Amy Klobuchar (D-MN), supported by other leading Representatives introduced the Breast Cancer Education and Awareness Requires Learning Young, *EARLY*, Act of 2009. The object of this Act is "to increase awareness of the risks of breast cancer in young women, and to provide support for those diagnosed with breast cancer." The bill has 260 co-sponsors, enough to guarantee passage by the House. However, the measure has stalled in the Senate.

The Bill met with a storm of protests by "experts in breast cancer prevention." These included Dr. Donald Berry, chairman of the Department of Biostatistics at the M.D. Anderson Cancer Center, who warned that the bill is misguided. "I leave politics to the politicians, why can't they leave science to the scientists? Except for family history, there are no important risks . . . for women younger than 40."

Dr. Leslie Bernstein, director of the City of Hope Comprehensive Cancer Center, also claimed that "We have no known environmental causes of breast cancer other than radiation . . . except when you are having a mammogram," a surprising and damaging admission.

However, these and other critics of EARLY are unaware of the scientific evidence on a wide range of avoidable causes of breast cancer. These include the Pill, estrogen replacement therapy, and living close to hazardous waste sites and nuclear plants.

Not surprisingly, the American Cancer Society (ACS), a strong proponent of routine premenopausal mammography, failed to comment on EARLY. In 1984, with its October flagship National Mammography Day, the ACS inaugurated the National Breast Cancer Awareness Month. This assured women that annual mammography starting at the age of 40 "results in a cure nearly 100 percent of the time." However, and still denied by the ACS, screening mammography poses significant dangers of radiation.

The routine practice of taking two films of each breast annually over 10 years, results in approximately 0.5 rad (radiation absorbed dose) exposure. This is about 500 times greater than exposure from a single chest X-ray, broadly focused on the entire chest rather than narrowly on the breast. Moreover, the premenopausal breast is highly sensitive to radiation. Each rad exposure increases risks of breast cancer by about 1%, with a cumulative 5% increased risk for each breast over a decade's screening. So, a premenopausal woman having annual mammograms over 10 years is exposed to roughly 5 rads. This is the approximate level of radiation received by a Japanese woman a mile or so away from where the Hiroshima or Nagasaki atom bombs were exploded.

Radiation risks are increased by fourfold for the 1% to 2% of women who may be unknowing and silent carriers of the A-T (ataxia-telangiectasia) gene, and thus highly sensitive to the carcinogenic effects of radiation. By some estimates, this accounts for up to 20% of all breast cancers diagnosed annually.

Of additional concern, missed cancers are common in premenopausal women due to the density of their breasts. Mammography also entails tight and often painful breast compression, particularly in premenopausal women. This may lead to the rupture of small blood vessels in or around small undetected breast cancers, and the lethal distant spread of malignant cells.

That most breast cancers are first recognized by women themselves was even admitted as early as 1985 by the American Cancer Society (ACS), the world's largest "non-profit" organization. At least 90 percent of women who develop breast cancer discover the tumors themselves."

As detailed in my 1999 publication in the prestigious *International Journal of Health Services*, the ACS is knee deep in conflicts of interest with the mammography industry. Five radiologists have served as ACS presidents and, in its every move, the ACS promotes the interests of the major manufacturers of mammogram machines and films, including Siemens, DuPont, General Electric, Eastman Kodak, and Piker. The mammography industry also conducts "research" for the ACS, to which it donates considerable funds. This blatant conflict of interest is hardly surprising. *The Chronicle of Philanthropy*, the world's leading charity watchdog, published a statement in 1993 that the ACS is "more interested in accumulating wealth than saving lives."

Not surprisingly, ACS promotion continues to lure women of all ages into mammography centers, leading them to believe that mammography is their best hope against breast cancer. An ACS communications director, questioned by journalist Kate Dempsey, admitted in an article published by the Massachusetts Women's Community's journal *Cancer*, "The ad isn't based on a study. When you make an advertisement, you just say what you can to get women in the door. You exaggerate a point . . . Mammography today is a lucrative [and] highly competitive business."

Furthermore, an analysis of several 1993 studies showed that women who regularly performed monthly breast self-examination (BSE) detected their cancers much earlier than those who failed to do so. However, the ACS and radiologists still claim that "no studies have clearly shown any benefit of BSE."

Apart from the importance of self-empowering women, the costs of BSE are trivial compared to the inflationary impact of mammography. The estimated annual costs for screening pre—and post-menopausal women are in excess of $10 billion, equivalent to about 14 percent of Medicare spending on prescription drugs. Costs of digital mammography, enthusiastically supported by radiologists and the radiology industry, are approximately four-fold greater, even in the absence of any evidence for its improved effectiveness.

Finally, and not surprisingly, premenopausal mammography is practiced by no nation other than the United States. As recently reported by the British journalist Liz Savage, "Earlier this year, *The Times of London* published a letter, signed by two dozen physicians and patient advocates, reprimanding the UK's National Health Service for not providing women with adequate information about the risks of screening mammography." The letter described "the harms associated with early detection of breast cancer by screening that are not widely acknowledged. The most important of these harms are over-diagnosis—and its frequent consequence, over-treatment."

ENDORSER:

Rosalie Bertell, PhD
Former President of the International Institute of Concern for Public Health, Toronto, Canada
Regent of the International Physicians for Humanitarian Medicine, Geneva, Switzerland

December 16, 2009

RECKLESS INDIFFERENCE OF THE AMERICAN CANCER SOCIETY TO CANCER PREVENTION

Early this month, top Republican Senator Charles E. Grassley sent letters to the American Cancer Society (ACS), besides the American Medical Association (AMA) and 31 other medical advocacy groups, asking them to provide detailed information on tax-deductible funds that they have received from drug and device makers. Such funds have encouraged these organizations to lobby on behalf of a wide range of industries and strongly influence public policy.

Senator Grassley also invited involvement of "whistleblowers interested in establishing communication regarding wrongdoing or misuse of public dollars." However, this wrongdoing still remains unrecognized by policy makers, let alone by the public. As a result, the incidence of a wide range of avoidable cancers has continued to escalate. Meanwhile, well-documented scientific information on their well-documented causes remains undisclosed or ignored by the ACS. (Epstein, S.S. Cancer Gate: How To Win The Losing Cancer War, 2005).

1971   The ACS refused to testify at Congressional hearings requiring FDA to ban the intramuscular injection of diethylstilbestrol, a synthetic estrogenic hormone, to fatten cattle, despite unequivocal evidence of its carcinogenicity, and the cancer risks of eating hormonal meat. Not surprisingly, U.S. meat is banned by other nations worldwide.

1977   The ACS opposed regulating black or dark brown hair dyes, based on paraphenylenediamine in spite of clear evidence of its risks of non-Hodgkins lymphoma, besides other cancers.

1978   Tony Mazzocchi, then senior international union labor representative, protested that "Occupational safety standards have received no support from the ACS." This has resulted in the increasing incidence of a wide range of avoidable cancers.

1978   Cong. Paul Rogers censured ACS for its failure to support the Clean Air Act in order to protect interests of the automobile industry

1982   The ACS adopted restrictive cancer policies, rejecting evidence based on standard rodent tests, which are widely accepted by governmental agencies worldwide and also by the International Agency for Research on Cancer.

1984   The ACS created the industry-funded October National Breast Cancer Awareness Month to falsely assure women that "early (mammography)

detection results in a cure nearly 100 percent of the time." Responding to question, ACS admitted: "Mammography today is a lucrative [and] highly competitive business." Also, the Awareness Month ignores substantial information on avoidable causes of breast cancer.

1992   The ACS supported the Chlorine Institute in defending the continued use of carcinogenic chlorinated pesticides, despite their environmental persistence and carcinogenicity.

1993   Anticipating the Public Broadcast Service (PBS) Frontline special "In Our Children's Food," the ACS trivialized pesticides as a cause of childhood cancer and charged PBS with "junk science." The ACS went further by questioning, "Can we afford the PBS?"

1994   The ACS published a highly flawed study designed to trivialize cancer risks from the use of dark hair dyes.

1998   The ACS allocated $330,000, under 1 percent of its then $680 million budget, to claimed research on environmental cancer.

1999   The ACS trivialized risks of breast, colon and prostate cancers from consumption of rBGH genetically modified milk. Not surprisingly, U.S. milk is banned by other nations worldwide.

2002   The ACS announced its active participation in the "Look Good . . . Feel Better Program," launched in 1989 by the Cosmetic Toiletry and Fragrance Association, to "help women cancer patients restore their appearance and self-image during chemotherapy and radiation treatment." This program was partnered by a wide range of leading cosmetics industries, which failed to disclose information on the carcinogenic, and other toxic ingredients in their products donated to unsuspecting women.

2002   The ACS reassured the nation that carcinogenicity exposures from dietary pesticides, "toxic waste in dump sites, "ionizing radiation from "closely controlled" nuclear power plants, and non-ionizing radiation, are all "at such low levels that cancer risks are negligible." ACS indifference to cancer prevention became embedded in national cancer policy, following the appointment of Dr. Andrew von Eschenbach, ACS Past President-Elect, as director of the National Cancer Institute (NCI).

2005   The ACS indifference to cancer prevention other than smoking, remains unchanged, despite the escalating incidence of cancer, and its $ billion budget.

Some of the more startling realities in the failure to prevent cancers are illustrated by their soaring increases from 1975 to 2005, when the latest NCI epidemiological data are available. These include:

- Malignant melanoma of the skin in adults has increased by 168 percent due to the use of sunscreens in childhood that fail to block long wave ultraviolet light;
- Thyroid cancer has increased by 124 percent due in large part to ionizing radiation;
- Non-Hodgkin's lymphoma has increased 76 percent due mostly to phenoxy herbicides; and phenylenediamine hair dyes;
- Testicular cancer has increased by 49 percent due to pesticides; hormonal ingredients in cosmetics and personal care products; and estrogen residues in meat;
- Childhood leukemia has increased by 55 percent due to ionizing radiation; domestic pesticides; nitrite preservatives in meats, particularly hot dogs; and parental exposures to occupational carcinogens;
- Ovary cancer (mortality) for women over the age of 65 has increased by 47 percent in African American women and 13 percent in Caucasian women due to genital use of talc powder;
- Breast cancer has increased 17 percent due to a wide range of factors. These include: birth control pills; estrogen replacement therapy; toxic hormonal ingredients in cosmetics and personal care products; diagnostic radiation; and routine premenopausal mammography, with a cumulative breast dose exposure of up to about five rads over ten years.

MAJOR CONFLICTS OF INTEREST

Public Relations

- 1998-2000: PR for the ACS was handled by Shandwick International, whose major clients included RJ Reynolds Tobacco Holdings.
- 2000-2002: PR for the ACS was handled by Edelman Public Relations, whose major clients included Brown & Williamson Tobacco Company, and the Altria Group, the parent company of Philip Morris, Kraft, and fast-food and soft drink beverage companies. All these companies were promptly dismissed once this information was revealed by the Cancer Prevention Coalition.

Industry Funding

ACS has received contributions in excess of $100,000 from a wide range of "Excalibur Donors," many of whom continue to manufacture carcinogenic products. These include:

- Petrochemical companies (DuPont; BP; and Pennzoil)
- Industrial waste companies (BFI Waste Systems)
- Junk food companies (Wendy's International; McDonalds's; Unilever/Best Foods; and Coca-Cola)
- Big Pharma (AstraZenceca; Bristol-Myers Squibb; GlaxoSmithKline; Merck & Company; and Novartis)
- Biotech companies (Amgen; and Genentech)
- Cosmetic companies (Christian Dior; Avon; Revlon; Elizabeth Arden; and Estee Lauder)
- Auto companies (Nissan; General Motors)

Nevertheless, as reported in the December 8, 2009 New York Times, the ACS responded that it "holds itself to the highest standards of transparency and public accountability, and we look forward to working with Senator Grassley to provide the information he requested."

THE CHRONICLE OF PHILANTHROPY

As the nation's leading charity watch dog, the Chronicle has warned against the transfer of money from the public purse to private hands. It also published a statement that "The ACS is more interested in accumulating wealth than in saving lives."

A copy of this release has been sent to Senator Charles E. Grassley, of Iowa.

May 7, 2010

AMERICAN CANCER SOCIETY TRIVIALIZES CANCER RISKS: BLATANT CONFLICTS OF INTEREST

The May 6 report by the President's Cancer Panel is well-documented. It warns of scientific evidence on avoidable causes of cancer from exposure to carcinogens in air, water, consumer products, and the workplace. It also warns of hormonal risks from exposure to Bisphenol-A (BPA) and other toxic plastic contaminants, says Samuel S. Epstein, M.D., Chairman of the Cancer Prevention Coalition (CPC).

Concerns on avoidable causes of cancer have been summarized in a January 23, 2009 Cancer Prevention Coalition press release, endorsed by 20 leading scientists and public policy experts, who urged that President Obama's cancer plan should prioritize prevention. These concerns were further detailed in a June 15, 2009 press release. Warnings of the risks of BPA are also detailed in a May 6, 2010 CPC release.

Some of the more startling realities in the National Cancer Institute's (NCI) and the "non-profit" American Cancer Society's (ACS) long-standing failure to prevent a very wide range of cancers are illustrated by their soaring increases from 1975 to 2005.

These include:

- Malignant melanoma of the skin in adults has increased by 168 percent due to the use of sunscreens in childhood that fail to block long wave ultraviolet light;
- Thyroid cancer has increased by 124 percent due in large part to ionizing radiation;
- Non-Hodgkin's lymphoma has increased 76 percent due mostly to phenoxy herbicides; and phenylenediamine hair dyes;
- Testicular cancer has increased by 49 percent due to pesticides; hormonal ingredients in cosmetics and personal care products; and estrogen residues in meat;
- Childhood leukemia has increased by 55 percent due to ionizing radiation; domestic pesticides; nitrite preservatives in meats, particularly hot dogs; and parental exposures to occupational carcinogens;
- Ovary cancer (mortality) for women over the age of 65 has increased by 47 percent in African American women and 13 percent in Caucasian women due to genital use of talc powder;

- Breast cancer has increased 17 percent due to a wide range of factors. These include: birth control pills; estrogen replacement therapy; toxic hormonal ingredients in cosmetics and personal care products; diagnostic radiation; and routine premenopausal mammography, with a cumulative breast dose exposure of up to about five rads over ten years.

Criticisms by the American Cancer Society that the President's Cancer Panel's report exaggerates avoidable cancer risks, reflect reckless indifference, besides narrow self-interest, warns Dr. Epstein.

In 1993, the nation's leading charity watch dog, *The Chronicle of Philanthropy*, warned against the transfer of money from the public purse to the private hands of the American Cancer Society. The Chronicle also published a statement that, "The ACS is more interested in accumulating wealth than saving lives."

These warnings are fully supported by the track record of the ACS for well over the last four decades.

- 1971: The ACS refused to testify at Congressional hearings requiring FDA to ban the intramuscular injection of diethylstilbestrol, a synthetic estrogenic hormone, to fatten cattle, prior to their entry into feedlots prior to slaughter, despite unequivocal evidence of its carcinogenicity, and the cancer risks of eating hormonal meat. Not surprisingly, U.S. meat is outlawed by most nations worldwide.
- 1977: The ACS opposed regulating black or dark brown hair dyes, based on paraphenylenediamine, in spite of clear evidence of its risks of non-Hodgkins lymphoma, besides other cancers.
- 1978: Tony Mazzocchi, then senior international union labor representative, protested that "Occupational safety standards have received no support from the ACS." This has resulted in the increasing incidence of a wide range of avoidable cancers.
- 1978: Congressman Paul Rogers censured ACS for its failure to support the Clean Air Act in order to protect interests of the automobile industry.
- 1982: The ACS adopted restrictive cancer policies, rejecting evidence based on standard rodent tests, which are widely accepted by governmental agencies worldwide and also by the International Agency for Research on Cancer.
- 1984: The ACS created the industry-funded October National Breast Cancer Awareness Month to falsely assure women that "early

(mammography) detection results in a cure nearly 100 percent of the time." Responding to question, ACS admitted: "Mammography today is a lucrative [and] highly competitive business." Also, the Awareness Month ignores substantial information on avoidable causes of breast cancer.

- 1992: The ACS supported the Chlorine Institute in defending the continued use of carcinogenic chlorinated pesticides, despite their environmental persistence and carcinogenicity.
- 1993: Anticipating the Public Broadcast Service (PBS) Frontline special "In Our Children's Food," the ACS trivialized pesticides as a cause of childhood cancer and charged PBS with "junk science." The ACS went further by questioning, "Can we afford the PBS?"
- 1994: The ACS published a highly flawed study designed to trivialize cancer risks from the use of dark hair dyes.
- 1998: The ACS allocated $330,000, under 1 percent of its then $680 million budget, to claimed research on environmental cancer.
- 1999: The ACS trivialized risks of breast, colon and prostate cancers from consumption of rBGH genetically modified milk. Not surprisingly, U.S. milk is outlawed by most nations worldwide.
- 2002: The ACS announced its active participation in the "Look Good . . . Feel Better Program," launched in 1989 by the Cosmetic Toiletry and Fragrance Association, to "help women cancer patients restore their appearance and self-image following chemotherapy and radiation treatment." This program was partnered by a wide range of leading cosmetics industries, which recklessly, if not criminally, failed to disclose information on the carcinogenic, and other toxic ingredients in their products donated to unsuspecting women.
- 2002: The ACS reassured the nation that carcinogenicity exposures from dietary pesticides, "toxic waste in dump sites, "ionizing radiation from "closely controlled" nuclear power plants, and non-ionizing radiation, are all "at such low levels that cancer risks are negligible." ACS indifference to cancer prevention became further embedded in national cancer policy, following the appointment of Dr. Andrew von Eschenbach, ACS Past President-Elect, as NCI Director.
- 2005: The ACS indifference to cancer prevention other than smoking, remains unchanged, despite the escalating incidence of cancer, and its $ billion budget.

The ACS's indifference to cancer prevention also reflects major conflicts of interest with regard to public relations, Dr. Epstein emphasizes.

PUBLIC RELATIONS

1998-2000: PR for the ACS was handled by Shandwick International, whose major clients included RJ Reynolds Tobacco Holdings.

2000-2002: PR for the ACS was handled by Edelman Public Relations, whose major clients included Brown & Williamson Tobacco Company, and the Altria Group, the parent company of Philip Morris, Kraft, and fast food and soft drink beverage companies. All these companies were promptly dismissed once this information was revealed by the CPC.

INDUSTRY FUNDING

The ACS's indifference to cancer prevention reflects major industry funding. ACS has received contributions in excess of $100,000 from a wide range of "Excalibur Donors," many of whom continue to manufacture carcinogenic products, points out Dr. Epstein.

These include:

-
- Petrochemical companies (DuPont; BP; and Pennzoil)
- Industrial waste companies (BFI Waste Systems)
- Junk food companies (Wendy's International; McDonalds's; Unilever/ Best Foods; and Coca-Cola)
- Big Pharma (AstraZenceca; Bristol-Myers Squibb; GlaxoSmithKline; Merck & Company; and Novartis)
- Biotech companies (Amgen; and Genentech)
- Cosmetic companies (Christian Dior; Avon; Revlon; Elizabeth Arden; and Estee Lauder)
- Auto companies (Nissan; General Motors)

Nevertheless, warns Dr. Epstein, in spite of this long-standing track record of flagrant conflicts of interest, as reported in the December 8, 2009 New York Times, the ACS responded that it "holds itself to the highest standards of transparency and public accountability."

March 14, 2011

THE AMERICAN CANCER SOCIETY (ACS): "MORE INTERESTED IN ACCUMULATING WEALTH THAN SAVING LIVES

A report on the American Cancer Society (ACS), "More Interested In Accumulating Wealth Than Saving Lives" was released today. This report is authored by Dr. Samuel Epstein, chairman of the Cancer Prevention Coalition, and Emeritus professor of Environmental and Occupational Medicine at the University of Illinois School of Public Health, and endorsed by Congressman John Conyers Jr., Chairman of the House Judiciary Committee, and Quentin Young M.D., Chairman of the Health and Medicine Policy research Group, and Past President of the American Public Health Association.

The report traces the track record of the ACS, since its founding in 1913 by a group of oncologists and wealthy business men until this year. It documents the virtually exclusive priority of the ACS to the diagnosis and treatment of cancer, with indifference to prevention, other than that due to faulty personal lifestyle. Commonly known as "blame the victim," this excludes the very wide range of scientifically well-documented avoidable causes of cancer.

The ACS track record also clearly reflects frank conflicts of interest. About half the ACS board are clinicians, oncologists, surgeons, and radiologists, mostly with close ties to the National Cancer Institute (NCI). Many board members and their institutional colleagues apply to and obtain funding from both the ACS and the NCI. Substantial NCI funds also go to ACS directors who sit on key NCI committees. Although the ACS asks its board members to leave the room when others review their funding proposals, this is just a token formality. In this private club, easy access to funding is one of the perks, as the board routinely rubber-stamps approvals. A significant amount of ACS funding also goes to this extended membership. Frank conflicts of interest are also evident in many ACS priorities. These include policies on mammography, the National Breast Cancer Awareness campaign, and the pesticide and cancer drug industries. These conflicts extend to the virtual privatization of national cancer policy.

For instance the ACS has close connections to the mammography industry. Five radiologists have served as ACS presidents. In its every move, the ACS reflects the interests of the major manufacturers of mammography, films and machines. These include Siemens, DuPont, General Electric, Eastman Kodak, and Piker, which allocate considerable funds to the ACS.

ACS promotion still continues to lure women of all ages into mammography centers, leading them to believe that mammography is their best hope against breast cancer. An ACS advertisement in a leading Massachusetts newspaper featured a photograph of two women in their twenties that recklessly promised that early detection results in a cure "nearly 100 percent of the time." An ACS communications director, questioned by journalist Kate Dempsey, responded in an article published by the Massachusetts Women's Community's journal *Cancer*: "The ad isn't based on a study. When you make an advertisement, you just say what you can to get women in the door. You exaggerate a point. Mammography today is a lucrative [and] highly competitive business." However, the National Academy of Science has warned that the premenopausal breast is highly sensitive to radiation, and that annual mammography can increase risks of breast cancer by 10%. Furthermore, the US Preventive Task Force, supported by the National Breast Cancer Coalition, has recently recommended that routine mammography should be delayed until the age of 50 and practiced every 2 years subsequently until the age of 75.

The ACS has also had a strong relation with a wide range of industries, including the pesticide and cancer drug. Responding to concerns on risks on carcinogenic pesticides in food, the ACS responded "We have no cancer cases in which pesticide use was confirmed as the cause." Also referring to concerns on the multibillion dollar cancer drug industry sales, the ACS dismisses "unproven," non-patentable and minimally toxic alternatives. This claim however is in the striking contrast to its hidden conflicts of interest.

Public Relations

1998-2000: PR for the ACS was handled by Shandwick International, whose major clients included R.J. Reynolds Tobacco Holdings.

2000-2002: PR for the ACS was handled by Edelman Public Relations, whose major clients included Brown & Williamson Tobacco Company, and Altria Group, the parent company of Philip Morris, Kraft, and fast food and soft drink beverage companies. All these companies were preemptively dismissed once this information was revealed by the Cancer Prevention Coalition.

Industry Funding

ACS has receive contributions in excess of $100,000 from a wide range of "Excalibur Donors." Some of these companies were responsible for environmental pollution with carcinogens, while others manufactured and sold products containing toxic and carcinogenic ingredients. These include:

- Petrochemical companies (DuPont; BP; and Pennzoil)
- Industrial waste companies (BFI Waste Systems)

- Big Pharma (AstraZeneca; Bristol-Myers Squibb; GlaxoSmithKline; Merck & Company; and Novartis)
- Auto companies (Nissan; and General Motors)
- Cosmetic companies (Christian Dior; Avon; Revlon; and Elizabeth Arden)
- Junk food companies (Wendy's International; McDonalds's; Unilever/ Best Foods; and Coca-Cola)
- Biotech companies (Amgen; and Genentech)

Nevertheless, as reported in the December 8, 2009 *New York Times*, the ACS claimed that it "holds itself to the highest standards of transparency and public accountability." Of major concern is the reckless record of the ACS with regard to cancer prevention over the past four decades.

1971   When studies unequivocally proved that diethylstilbestrol (DES) caused vaginal cancers in teenage daughters of women administered the drug during pregnancy, the ACS refused an invitation to testify at Congressional hearings to require the Food and Drug Administration to ban its use as an animal feed additive. It gave no reason for its refusal. Not surprisingly, U.S. meat is banned by other nations worldwide.

1983   The ACS refused to join a coalition of the March of Dimes, American Heart Association, and the American Lung Association to support the Clean Air Act.

1992   The ACS issued a joint statement with the Chlorine Institute in support of the continued global use of organochlorine pesticides, despite clear evidence that some were known to cause breast cancer. In this statement, ACS vice president Clark Heath, M.D., dismissed the evidence of any risk as "preliminary and mostly based on a weak and indirect association."

1993   Just before PBS *Frontline* aired the special entitled, "In Our Children's Food," the ACS came out in support of the pesticide industry. In a damage-control memorandum sent to some 48 regional divisions and their 3,000 local offices, the ACS trivialized pesticides as a cause of childhood cancer. The ACS also reassured the public that carcinogenic pesticide residues in food are safe, even for babies.

1994   The ACS published a study designed to reassure women on the safety of dark permanent hair dyes, and to trivialize risk of fatal and non-fatal cancers, particularly non-Hodgkin lymphoma, as documented in over six prior reports.

1999   The ACS denied any risks of cancer from drinking genetically-engineered (rBGH) milk. Its position has remained unchanged in spite of strong scientific decade old strong evidence relating rBGH milk to major risks of breast, prostate, and colon cancers.

2000 The Washington-Insider *Cancer Letter*, revealed that the ACS has close ties to the tobacco industry, notably Shandwick International, representing R.J. Reynolds Tobacco Holdings, and subsequently Edelman Public Relations, representing Brown &Williamson Tobacco company.

2002 The ACS initiated the "Look Good . . . Feel Better" program to teach women cancer patients beauty techniques to help restore their appearance and self-image during chemotherapy and radiation treatment." This program was partnered by the National Cosmetology Association and The Cosmetic, Toiletry and Fragrance Association Foundation, which failed to disclose the wide range of carcinogenic ingredients in toiletries and cosmetics. These trade organizations also failed to disclose evidence of risks of breast and other cancers following long-term use of black or dark brown permanent and semi-permanent hair dyes. The ACS also failed to inform women of these avoidable risks. The Environmental Cancer Risk Section of the *ACS Facts and Figures Report* also reassured that carcinogenic exposures from dietary pesticides, "toxic wastes in dump sites"—are "all at such low levels that risks are negligible."

2007 The ACS indifference to cancer prevention, other than smoking, has remained unchanged despite its $1 billion budget, and despite the escalating incidence of cancer from 1975. This includes post menopausal breast cancer, 23%; childhood cancer, 30%; testis cancer 60%; and non-Hodgkin lymphoma, 82%.

2009 The ACS budget was about $1 billion, of which 17% was allotted to smoking cessation programs, and 28% to support services and salaries. The top three executive salaries ranged from $670,000 to $1.2 million.

2010 The ACS rejected the April 2010 President's Cancer Panel report, "Reducing Environmental Cancer." This had been widely endorsed by leading scientific and public policy experts. Nevertheless, the ACS brazenly claimed that more studies were needed to justify this conclusion.

The ACS track record of frank indifference to cancer prevention, other than that due to faulty lifestyle, extends to cancer organizations in Canada and 90 nations worldwide in support of their "Relay For Life" programs. Team members take turns to walk or run around a track for 12-24 hours. "Through the Relay, these organizations bring together passionate volunteers, to take action in the international movement to end cancer," by stopping smoking and developing healthy lifestyles. Funds raised by these Relays support local organizations' cancer control programs, services, and research." These organizations also contribute part of their funds to ACS "cancer control programs" worldwide.

Clearly the ACS continues to forfeit the decades old international public trust and support.

APPENDIX A

THE STOP CANCER BEFORE IT STARTS CAMPAIGN: HOW TO WIN THE LOSING WAR AGAINST CANCER

SPONSORS AND ENDORSERS

February 2003

SPONSORS

Nicholas Ashford, PhD, JD,
Professor, Technology and Policy, Massachusetts Institute of Technology,
Member, Governing Board (Massachusetts) Alliance for a Healthy Tomorrow,
    and CPC Board of Directors
nashford@mit.edu

Kenny Ausubel,
President, Bioneers, and the Collective Heritage Institute
kenny@bioneers.org

Barry Castleman, PhD,
Environmental Consultant, and
CPC Board of Directors
bcastleman@earthlink.net

Edward Goldsmith, MA,
Publisher, The Ecologist, and CPC Board of Directors
teddy.goldsmith@virgin.net

JeffreyHollender,
President, Seventh Generation
jeffrey@seventhgeneration.com

Anthony Mazzocchi
Founder of The Labor Party, and Member of the Debs-Jones-Douglass Labor
    Institute, and CPC Board of Directors

Horst M. Rechelbacher,
Founder, Aveda
Corporation, and President, Intelligent Nutrients
horst@intelligentnutrients.com

Quentin Young, MD, Chairman, Health and Medicine Policy
Research Group, National Coordinator of the Physicians for a National Health
    Program
Past President of the American Public Health Association, and CPC Board
    of Directors
quentin@pnhp.org

ENDORSEMENTS
Winfield J. Abbe, PhD
Former Associate Professor Physics, University of Georgia
Cancer prevention activist, Athens, GA
wjabbe@aol.com

Thomas J. Barnard, MD, CCFP, FAAFP
Adjunct Professor of Family Medicine, University of Western Ontario, Canada
Adjunct Professor of Human Biology and Nutritional Sciences, University of
    Guelph, Ontario, Canada
barnard@mnsi.net

Maude Barlow
National Chairperson, The Council of Canadians, Ottawa, Ontario, Canada
Director, International Forum on Globalization
mbarlow8965@rogers.com

Gregor Barnum
Executive Director, The Household Toxins Institute, Burlington, VT
gregor@seventhgeneration.com

Rosalie Bertell, PhD
President, International Institute of Concern for Public Health, Toronto,
    Canada
rosaliebertell@greynun.org

Brent Blackwelder, PhD
President, Friends of the Earth, Washington, D.C.
bblackwelder@foe.org

Judy Brady
GreenAction, and Toxic Links Coalition, San Francisco, CA
Member, CPC Board of Directors
jibasmil@aol.com

Elaine Broadhead
Environmental Activist, Middlesburg, VA
elainebroadhead@yahoo.com

James Brophy
Occupational Health Clinics for Ontario Workers, Ontario, Canada
jimbrophy@yahoo.com

Chris Busby, PhD, MRSC
Scientific Secretary, European Committee on Radiation Risks
Member, UK Government Committee on Radiation Risk for Internal Emitters,
    and UK Ministry of Defense
Oversight Committee on Depleted Uranium
christo@greenaudit.org

Leopoldo Caltagirone, PhD
Chairman, Division of Biological Control, Berkeley, CA
lcbiocon@berkeley.edu

Liane Casten
Publisher, Chicago Media Watch, Chicago, IL
lcasten@sbcglobal.net

L. Terry Chappell, MD
President, The International College of Integrative Medicine, Bluffton, OH
terrychappell@blogspot.com

Richard Clapp, MPH, DSc
Professor of Public Health, Boston University School of Public Health, Boston, MA
Member, Governing Board (Massachusetts) Alliance for a Healthy Tomorrow
richard.clapp@gmail.com

Gary Cohen
Executive Director, Environmental Health Fund, Jamaica Plain, MA
Director, Health Care Without Harm
gcohen@hcwh.org

Paul Connett, PhD
Professor of Chemistry, St. Lawrence University, Canton, NY
President, Fluoride Action Network
paul@fluoridealert.org

Mary Cook
Managing Director, Occupational Health Clinics for Ontario Workers (OHCOW), Ontario, Canada
cook@ohcow.on.ca

Ronnie Cummins
National Director, Organic Consumers Association, Little Marais, MN
ronnie@organicconsumers.org

Alexandra Delinick, MD
Dean, School of Homeopathic Therapy, Vassil Levsky University, Sofia, Bulgaria
(Past, General Secretary, International Medical Homeopathic League)
homandgv@hol.gr

Lynn Ehrle, MEd
Senior Research Fellow, CPC, Plymouth, MI
Vice President, Consumers Alliance of Michigan
ehrlebird@organicconsumers.org

Anwar Fazal
Chairperson, World Alliance for Breastfeeding Action
Senior Regional Advisor, the Urban Governance Initiative and United Nations
    Development Programme, Kuala
Lumpur, Malaysia
Right Livelihood Award Laureate (The Alternative Nobel Prize)
(Former President, International Organization of Consumers Union)
anwarfazal2004@yahoo.com

Michael Green
Executive Director, Center for Environmental Health, Oakland, CA
ceh@cehca.org

Lennart Hardell, MD, PhD
Professor Epidemiology, University Hospital, Umea, Sweden
lennart.hardell@orebroll.se

James Huff, PhD
National Institute of Environmental Health Sciences, Research Triangle
    Park, NC
huff1@niehs.nih.gov

Alison Linnecar
Coordinator, International Baby Food Action Network (IBFAN-GIFA)
Right Livelihood Award Laureate (The Alternative Nobel Prize)
alison.linnecar@gifa.org

Joseph Mangano, MPH, MBA
National Coordinator, Radiation and Public Health Project, Brooklyn, NY
odiejoe@aol.com

Elizabeth May
Director, Sierra Club of Canada, Ottawa, Canada
leader@greenparty.ca

Vicki Meyer, PhD
Faculty, Women's Health, DePaul University, Chicago, IL
Founder, International Organization to Reclaim Menopause
vmeyer@depaul.edu

Raúl Montenegro, PhD
Professor Evolutionary Biology, University Cordoba, Argentine
President, FUNAM (Foundation for Environmental Defense)
raulmontenegro@flash.com.ar

Vicente Navarro, MD
Professor of Health and Public Policy, The Johns Hopkins University, Baltimore, MD
Professor of Political and Social Sciences, Universitat Pompeu Fabra, Spain
Editor-in-Chief, International Journal of Health Services
vnavarro@jhsph.edu

Peter Orris, MD, MPH
Professor, Occupational Medicine, University of Illinois Medical School, Chicago, IL
Professor, Internal and Preventive Medicine, Rush Medical College, Chicago, IL
Professor, Preventive Medicine, Northwestern University Feinberg School of Medicine, Chicago, IL
porris@uic.edu

Marjorie Roswell
Environmental activist, Baltimore, MD
mroswell@gmail.com

Janette Sherman, MD
Consultant Toxicologist, Alexandria, VA
Research Associate, Radiation and Public Health Project, NY
toxdoc.js@verizon.net

Ernest Sternglass, PhD
Professor Emeritus, Department of Radiology, University of Pittsburgh, Pittsburgh, PA
erneststernglass@twcny.rr.com

Daniel Teitelbaum, MD
Professor, Preventive Medicine, University of Colorado, Denver, CO
toxdoc@ix.netcom.com

Stephen Tvedten, TIPM, CEI
Director, Institute of Pest Management, Inc., Marne, MI
stvedten@att.net

Jakob von Uexkull
President, Right Livelihood Award Foundation, Stockholm, Sweden
jakob@worldfuturecouncil.org

CPSIA information can be obtained at www.ICGtesting.com
Printed in the USA
LVOW112001230512

283009LV00001B/318/P